Brainwash Yourself
THIN

*Reclaim the power to create the life
and body you deserve*

Lindis Courtney

Recommendations

"*Brainwash Yourself Thin* is a much-needed manual for a world that lives to excess. Many of us have been out of touch with our emotions for as long as we can remember and mindlessly turn to food to comfort ourselves and fill the void. This book is a realistic manual that will help you to unlearn years of this negative behavior. I highly recommend this as a vital tool for permanently changing and taking control of your life!"

—*Taylor LeBaron, author, Cutting Myself in Half: 150 pounds lost, one byte at a time*

"I would not hesitate to recommend Lindis to anyone who wants to make change in their life. Her incisive questions and comments pushed me to reevaluate long-held belief systems that I didn't even know existed. After years of trying seemingly every diet and exercise program, I thought there was nothing I could do to lose weight. It was only after working with Lindis that I realized that it wasn't simply a thought. It was something much more powerful; it was a belief system. Within three months of working with Lindis, I began running (something I *never* imagined doing) and eating healthier. By the end of the three months, I had lost 15 pounds, gone down a dress size and am in the best shape I've been in since high school. I can't thank Lindis enough for all her help and support!"

—*Lauren Y., lawyer, Virginia*

"Lindis has been invaluable to me in helping me uncover my lack of commitment to my health goals. She helped me set realistic goals, which would help me to not be on a 'diet,' but have a lifestyle change. She helped me become aware of my relationship with food. She challenged me to make the hard decisions. She has set me on a path of positive change and commitment, and now, six months down the road, I still exercise regularly, am aware of what I'm eating and have lost 11 kilos!"

—*M.D. project director, in India*

"Lindis is a wonderful person! She is not only professional and extremely knowledgeable in her subject, but she is a partner by your side to make your personal goals happen! Besides having the goal to live a healthy life, I came to Lindis with the desire to write my first book. Not only did she understand how important that step was for me, but she also helped me along the way to bring it to completion. I am forever thankful to her for accompanying me on this path, and I would recommend her unreservedly any time!"

—*Anja Serfontein, life coach, ahealthylifewithchocolate.wordpress.com, Taiwan*

Lindis Courtney Coaching & Development
Gamleveien 87
Sandnes
Norway

www.lindiscourtney.com

DISCLAIMER

This book is not intended to replace medical advice or to be a substitute for a physician or psychologist/therapist/counselor. All the information contained herein, is the sole opinion of the author. Results will vary for each individual who follows the recommendations. Always seek the advice of a professional before beginning any weight-loss or exercise program. The author and publisher specifically disclaim any and all liability arising from the use of any information contained in this book. If you are under the care of a physician or other medical or psychological professional, he or she can advise you about the information described in this book.

The privacy of individuals mentioned in this book has been protected by changing their names and any identifying details. In addition, certain people and events have been crafted to illustrate important points.

This book is dedicated to you.

"If one advances confidently in the direction of his dreams, and endeavors to live the life that he has imagined, he will meet with a success unexpected in common hours."

—Henry David Thoreau, American philosopher (1817-1862)

Contents

The Power of
Positive Brainwashing

Brainwash Yourself Thin is one of the most important books you'll ever read on weight loss. It's the missing link between your desire for a lean body and your ability to achieve it. You and the entire Western world already know what to do (eat right and exercise), but you haven't figured out how to make yourself do it.

So, what stops you from taking the right actions to attain your dream body? You do! You're the culprit. Why? Because you have a mental blueprint filled with debilitating beliefs, thoughts and emotions that keep you overweight. This subconscious driving force defines who you are, how you think, what you believe, what you habitually do, and how you typically feel about yourself. It determines your success in life, both on and off the bathroom scale. If you don't break down and rebuild this mental blueprint, you'll never achieve a lean and healthy body. But if you do, you can become thin and stay there.

I call this book *Brainwash Yourself Thin* because at some point in your life you became brainwashed fat, and this, my dear friend, needs to be reversed. You've been brainwashed to believe that eating the cookie will make you feel better. You've been brainwashed to believe that achieving your ideal weight is impossible or that being thin means deprivation.

You've been brainwashed to believe you're powerless and unworthy. None of this is true, but because you believe it, you provide the evidence to convict yourself.

The battle of the bulge is really a battle of the mind. All day every day, you think thoughts and experience feelings you're not aware of. In fact, an estimated 45,000 thoughts go through your head each day, and 95 percent of them are repeated from the day before! Let's say you step on the scale and the reading is 3 pounds higher than what it was last week. "I'm never going to lose weight," you think. You go to the kitchen looking for consolation and grab a chocolate muffin. "What's the point of trying to eat healthy anyway?" you think. "Dieting doesn't work." You head to the mall and try on five different outfits. They are all too tight. "I'm such a failure," you think. "What's wrong with me? Why can't I lose weight?" On the way out, you buy a candy bar to comfort you on the ride home. "I need this," you think.

The thoughts constantly running through your head define who you are mentally, emotionally and even physically. They drive your decision-making and, in turn, your actions. For many people, the result is excess pounds, but it doesn't have to be that way. You can break the cycle by guiding your thoughts. Most likely, you have never been taught *how* to think, so you are not aware of your own power to steer your thoughts in the direction you want to go.

So in essence, reaching goal weight and staying there is a mind game. Think the right thoughts on a daily basis and you'll take the right actions. Win the mind game and you can become forever thin. Lose the mind game and you keep the body you have now.

Brainwash Yourself Thin works because it exposes your unhealthy thoughts and limiting beliefs and exchanges them for powerful thoughts and beliefs that support your goals and efforts. Then and only then are you ready to receive my eating and exercise recommendations that take the mystery out of weight loss. The self-analysis you undergo while reading this book is an enlightenment process that will affect you on the following levels:

- **Raised Consciousness**. You will gain awareness of your food addiction and the consequences thereof, so that you are psychologically motivated to make intelligent choices about what you need and want in life.

- **Emotional Arousal.** You will become so emotionally aroused (excited, frustrated, exasperated) that you will be brave enough to break through your obstacles.

- **Self-Reevaluation.** You will observe your thoughts and actions like an undercover agent and evaluate them. Discovering why you do what you do will empower you to throw out useless thoughts and behaviors.

- **Renewal of Commitment**. You will accept your responsibility for what occurred in the past and renew your commitment to what you can do with your present and future.

- **Re-patterned Habits.** You will throw out addictive behaviors and negative thinking and eagerly and willingly create healthy new patterns that will give you long-lasting joy.

- **Discovery of Your Unique Purpose.** You will become mentally and physically empowered to discover, pursue, and carry out your true purpose in life.

In essence, *Brainwash Yourself Thin* teaches you how to raise your level of awareness of what's standing in the way of the life and body you desire, and it shows you how to remove these mental obstacles.

Most change experts agree that permanent change occurs via six stages: pre-contemplation (resisting change), contemplation (weighing options), preparation (getting ready), action (taking small steps), maintenance (staying strong) and termination (when change is permanent).

If you skip a stage or two, your chances for success are limited, so *Brainwash Yourself Thin* diligently guides you through the comprehensive six-step change process. By reading each page of this book and doing the self-awareness exercises, you'll gradually be brainwashed thin. Your newfound commitment will fuel the process of creating your unique road map to the life and body of your dreams.

Your perspective on yourself, your life, and your potential to reach your target weight will change. By the end of the book, you'll be embarking on a new way of eating that can lead to consistent weight loss. You'll be in the driver's seat, and you will make decisions that move you closer and closer to your goals.

No matter what your story is, no matter how long you've battled with overeating or eating unhealthily, you can reach goal weight and stay there. Through my own experiences and watching those of countless others, I have come to realize that when you're willing to be unblocked, the solution presents itself and the pounds are released. When the student is willing to learn, the teacher miraculously appears.

My Story

So, who am I? Have I always been thin? I wish! My weight battle started in boarding school. No, it wasn't some fancy rich girl's prep school in New England. My teenage years were spent at a co-ed Christian boarding school in a small farming town in Minnesota.

My earliest years had been spent far from there, in New York City. My parents were loving yet dysfunctional. My dad was an alcoholic, and he and my mom fought a lot, so there was a lot of anger along with the joy. But there wasn't much communication. It seemed okay to yell or to laugh, but any other emotion was ignored or rebuked. I couldn't approach my parents about their fighting or things that bothered me at school or problems I had with friends. So I shut myself off from those feelings and went about my business.

When I was 14, my mom had had enough and left, divorcing my dad and moving back to Norway, where she'd grown up. My older brother and sister had already moved out, so it was just me and my dad. There I was in Brooklyn, fourteen years old, cooking and cleaning and abiding by what I considered to be ridiculously strict curfews. So I found a way out. I convinced him that attending a Christian boarding school would be a great experience for me, and off I went to the farmlands of the Midwest.

On the outside, it appeared that I was a well-adjusted teenager, thriving in my new social setting. On the inside, I had a lot of insecurities that I didn't know how to deal with. Food became an effective way to distract me and comfort me when I was lonely. It seemed harmless enough to join a bunch of giggling teenage girls to pig out on chocolate, chips, and ice cream. To reduce the damage, we would diet and then binge, eating like crazy for a week and then starve it off the week after. And so the yo-yo cycle began.

In college, the overeating habit continued to grow in size and frequency. By the time I entered the workforce, my addiction was literally full blown.

My daily routine was very predictable. I would eat a small breakfast in the morning and a normal-sized lunch at work with friends. But when I finally got home, it was full feast. I would have dinner, and then be "hungry" an hour later and look for snacks. I buried my feelings of insecurity in pasta. I celebrated my short-lived victories of promotions and awards with Oreos. My anger was subdued by ravaging a bag of Nachos. Each evening I was eating three or four times after dinner just to numb myself from the day's stress! I'd eat until I was very full or just couldn't eat any more. Food was basically my sedative that put me to sleep each evening.

For more than three decades, food remained my drug of choice even though I desperately wanted to be thin. I tried every diet and starvation plan, gaining and losing according to my emotional state. At my worst, I weighed 200 pounds when the healthy-weight chart said I should weigh 145.

All the while, you could say that I appeared to be successful. I climbed corporate ladders to fatten my bank account and build my self-esteem. My achievements of fancier titles and bigger paychecks, however, provided only fleeting moments of happiness. I still used food to celebrate my short-lived victories, calm my anxieties, and numb my insecurities. I was dissatisfied with my work and my personal life, and my reliance on food and my quest for more money kept me from discovering what would truly make me happy.

In 2009, I hit rock bottom. I wanted to be a perfect mother who managed home life and corporate life with wit and charm. Instead, I was a stressed-out emotional wreck and 40 pounds overweight. I finally got honest with myself. My life and my weight were out of control. I wanted to lose the food addiction and eat like a *normal* person, without struggle and without deprivation. I wanted my life to make sense and for it to be fulfilling on an emotional, spiritual and physical level.

All my life, I had been encouraging—sometimes badgering—friends, family members and even taxi drivers to let go of the past, discover their passions, and go out into the world to achieve their dreams. But I wasn't practicing what I preached.

That changed in 2009, when I walked away from my corporate career and completed a professional life coaching certification with over 125 hours of classes that blew my mind. I started to see how positive brainwashing (changing your beliefs to serve you), coupled with the pursuit of a compelling purpose, was my ticket out of food addiction. Little by little, I started to break down my negative mental blueprint and rebuild it layer by layer with positive truths that pushed me forward.

The more I learned about myself and experienced the amazing results of positive brainwashing, the more certain I was about what I wanted to do with my life: I was born to be a weight-loss coach who motivated and inspired others to let go of their disempowering mental blueprints so they could freely pursue their unique purposes in life.

Brainwash Yourself Thin is a system for food-addiction recovery. If you knowingly and willingly overeat or binge and yet desperately long to be thin, you're a food addict. You misuse food to the point that it causes you emotional and physical pain. *Brainwash Yourself Thin* will help you achieve your goal weight and stay thin because it will expose and address your addiction head-on. This is the same system I used to lose 40 pounds and keep it off.

Willpower is trying everything under the sun until you achieve what you want to achieve. My "everything under the sun" was researching the best experts in the field of personal development and weight loss to create this recovery system. I wanted to find a cure for my food addiction and I found it.

These are the underlying principles of the *Brainwash Yourself Thin* strategy:

 # 1 You must get yourself mentally ready for change. Most people fail to change because they don't mentally psyche themselves up and prepare for it. *Brainwash Yourself Thin* is structured around six stages of change that are the industry standard for overcoming addiction. As you travel through each stage, you bolster your determination to take steps toward recovery.

 # 2 You must think in ways that get you the results that you want in life. Your mind steers your life. If you think you can, you can. If you think you'll fail, you'll fail. Your thoughts determine your reality and define you. "As a man thinketh in his heart, so is he" (Proverbs 23:7). I'll show you how to adapt new beliefs and thought habits that can redefine you and change the course of your life.

 # 3 You must meet your six basic human needs. Your biggest driving force in life is your desire to meet your six basic human needs. Food addicts try to meet these needs with food, but you will learn to meet them by pursuing your purpose, growing spiritually, relishing in nurturing relationships, and embracing a healthy lifestyle.

 # 4 You must follow a predictable pattern of eating that gives you variety, taste, and consistent weight loss all the way to goal weight, and you must exercise efficiently.

For the first time in my life, weight loss is no longer a mystery. I finally understand the science of nutrition and exercise. I now know what, when, and how much to eat to achieve and maintain goal weight. I also have formed a completely different outlook and approach to exercise. In the past, dieting and exercise were torture without any benefit. Now, eating right and exercising is a joyous affair with solid results. I'll help you kick-start your own incredible transformation in the first few weeks.

 # 5 You must have a coach, accountability partner, or support group to motivate you and hold you accountable.

If you could have reached goal weight on your own, you would have done it by now. I spent 30 years being overweight because I was trying to do it alone. Once I committed to changing, I sought out the services of a weight-loss behavioral specialist to hold me accountable, challenge my faulty thinking, and inspire me to think "success." Hiring a coach or joining a support group is one of the most important steps you can take to set in motion your new mind-set and your new body.

It's because of my research, personal experience, and two years of training as a certified professional life coach that I was able to compile this book for you. Anyone with the motivation and the perseverance to break free from addiction can adapt the *Brainwash Yourself Thin* strategy to achieve success both on and off the scale.

The Key Success Factor of Transformation

Brainwash Yourself Thin has been deliberately compiled into an interactive book that you *do* rather than a typical book that you *read*. That's because the key factor of becoming forever thin is the wisdom and self-enlightenment you derive from doing the interactive challenges interspersed throughout these pages. When you openly and honestly expose and evaluate your life, your beliefs, and your habits (the good, the bad *and* the ugly), you suddenly see things that scream to be changed. Aspects of your life that you have tolerated for years suddenly are no longer acceptable. In fact, they need to be changed immediately! You demand more from yourself and boldly go about making it happen. You become driven and passionate about what you really want to achieve in your lifetime.

So take advantage of all the interactive assessments and questions in this book. The magic of your recovery lies in your discovery of what your responses mean to you and, equally important, what you're going to do about them. So you'll want to hold on to your responses to the written exercises for regular review and reflection. You can grab a notebook and pen or download a complimentary workbook that includes all of the written exercises contained in this book at www.lindiscourtney.com (on the coaching page, under "tools"). Do it right now so you have it in your hands from the start.

Let me take this opportunity to thank you for going with me on this journey to unlock the door to a happier and healthier life. While you're at my website, take a minute to join my community to receive inspiration and guidance for a life of power and purpose.

The Six Stages of Permanent Change

How many times have you looked in the mirror and vowed, "I'm going to lose this weight once and for all"? You join a gym, throw out (or eat) all the Oreos in the house, and vow to eat only soup, salad, and cereal for the next month. This strategy doesn't last long, does it? Within a few days (or hours), you're back in the cookie jar. Why? According to change experts, you weren't ready for change. You skipped two important steps that need to be completed *before* you can go into action mode: contemplation and preparation. Without taking those steps, it's sort of like jumping into battle without assessing your strategy, the enemy's capabilities, the skill set of your team, and the effectiveness of your weapons. You were set up for failure from the get-go.

Think about some major life changes you've experienced, like getting married, moving across the country, buying a home, having kids, starting a business, or taking a big trip. In most of these situations, you prepared yourself mentally, financially, emotionally and logistically. But when you decided to change your whole way of eating, you hopped right into action mode as if it was going to be a walk in the park. Then when you failed again for the umpteenth time, you beat yourself up: "What's wrong with me? It should have been so simple."

Well, weight loss is not so simple. Otherwise, you'd already be your ideal size. It doesn't have to brain surgery either. You just have to embrace your weight-loss project like any other major event in your life: Prepare for it mentally, physically, and emotionally and gather experts to assist you along the way.

Brainwash Yourself Thin will lead you on a magical journey through the six stages of change so that you can reach your goal weight and stay there. It's magical because it affects you on both unconscious and conscious levels. Your resistance to change will slowly dissipate. Each phase of the process will raise your awareness, prepare you to accept responsibility, and emotionally motivate you to take action.

This is the exact six-step process I used for my recovery from food addiction. I had been trying to lose 40 pounds for over 30 years with no success. But once I committed to this path, the weight fell off. The invisible walls of addiction that had imprisoned me for decades evaporated. You can experience the same breakthrough by traveling through the six stages of change.

The Six Stages of Change

According to Prochaska, Norcross, and DiClementi (1995), the change process involves six progressive stages of readiness.[1] To illustrate each stage, let's examine how Marissa, a 35-year-old sales manager from Ohio, develops through the change process.

(1) **Pre-Contemplation**: Marissa is 45 pounds overweight, but she isn't ready to change; she's in denial about her problem.

When confronted by her family members about her weight, she brushes them off, saying, "I just have a large frame. I always have."

(2) **Contemplation**: In the second stage of change, Marissa begins to acknowledge that there's a problem. Her clothes feel tighter and she feels frustrated when she catches a glimpse of herself in a mirror. She contemplates making small changes. "I need to cut down on Coke" or "I should eat less takeout food."

(3) **Preparation**: Marissa admits that she's overweight and that she needs to do something about it. She says, "I'm going to hire a weight-loss coach," or, "I'll join Weight Watchers." Even though Marissa communicates her desire to change and plans an action step, she still may only be in the talking-about-it phase. She may be waiting on more information or inspiration before committing to taking a positive step.

(4) **Action:** Marissa throws out all the junk food in her house, hires a weight-loss coach, and starts writing down everything she eats each day. Not all her efforts are perfect, but she's actively trying new strategies and making small attempts to change.

(5) **Maintenance and Relapse:** Marissa is mastering the change process. She is no longer binging or overeating. She enjoys healthy eating and regular exercise. She feels confident about what to do to maintain her weight loss. That's not to say she won't relapse and fall back into overeating—relapse can occur at any stage in the process. But if Marissa goes off track, she knows what to do to get back on it. If her recovery from overeating is successful, she'll choose to continue with the maintenance stage and her chance of relapse will grow smaller and smaller.

(6) **Termination**: This stage is true victory. Marissa has reached her goal weight and maintained it for some time. She no longer feels at risk of going back to her old ways. She has learned new ways to tackle the ups and downs of life without food. Eating well and exercising regularly are her preferred way of life.

This is not a perfect journey. Like Marissa, most people will "recycle" through the stages of change several times before the change becomes fully established. Trying and failing give you better odds of success than if you didn't try at all. Any action, even the wrong action, is better than no action.

Take a moment to reflect on where you are in your change cycle. Do you think you can hop over the first two steps and jump into action mode? No, you can't. Start at the beginning. You may discover some things about yourself and your relationship to food that you weren't aware of. This will strengthen your desire to reach your goal weight and keep you motivated.

STAGES	CHARACTERISTICS
Pre-Contemplation: *Resisting change*	Are you in denial about your food addiction? Have you given up on having a leaner body?
Contemplation: *Sitting on the fence*	Are you exploring the pros and cons of changing? Do you burn with desire to reach goal weight?
Preparation: *Getting ready*	Are you at the point where you are willing to experiment with small changes? Are you ready to create a plan?
Action: *Time to move*	Are you actively making changes to your eating and exercise habits? Are you learning by doing?
Maintenance and Relapse Prevention: *Keeping strong*	Are you maintaining the positive new behavior and seeing results?
Termination: *Second nature*	Do eating healthily and exercising regularly feel comfortable? Is it your preferred way of life?

What stage are you in?

What makes you believe you're at that stage?

Pre-Contemplation

"Me, a Food Addict?"

CHARACTERISTICS OF PRE-CONTEMPLATION	HELPFUL STRATEGIES
• Denial	• Assess yourself
• Excuses	• Learn about the problem
• Uninterested, unaware, unwilling	• Weigh the risks vs. rewards
	• Focus on the positive outcomes of change

"It isn't that they can't see the solution.
It is that they can't see the problem."
—G.K. Chesterton

Defining Characteristics of the Pre-contemplation Stage

If you're in the pre-contemplation stage, you probably don't even want to read this book. You're not really interested in changing your intimate relationship with food. You may be downright opposed to changing, or you may just want to postpone it until the distant future. You may have tried to lose weight and keep it off so many times that you've lost hope.

If you're knee-deep in your food addiction, it might be hard to imagine yourself ever climbing out of it. This chapter will raise your awareness about your unhealthy relationship to food and shine a light on your body and weight issues. You'll move along a continuum from unconscious, unaware, and unwilling to conscious, aware and willing to change. A small mustard seed of motivation will also be planted by highlighting the personal benefits of eating right and exercising regularly.

Be warned, this chapter may feel like an unwanted intervention or a big waste of time. You'll resist doing the exercises. Your responses to the questions may depress you. You may get mad at me for asking them. You may feel more hopeless about your situation than before. Uncomfortable feelings might emerge that you would rather avoid. But trust the process and stay out of the kitchen! The key to a good intervention is that when it's over, your honest appraisal of yourself opens you up to making a change. Remember, you can become forever thin if you successfully travel through these stages. Trust the process.

Assess Yourself

"We make ourselves real by telling the truth."
—**Thomas Merton**

Are You in Denial?

In an alcoholic family, denial is the "pink elephant" sitting in the middle of the living room that no one acknowledges. Dad may be drunk and falling off his chair, but everyone pretends not to see it. For food addicts, denial is pretending that you don't have a problem or that the problem isn't your fault. A statement I hear often from prospective clients is, "I hardly eat at all. I don't know why I'm this size." When confronted by family and friends about their overeating, those in denial might say, "I don't care about what other people think—I like my size," or, "I'm not addicted to food—I can give up snacks any time I want."

If you're in denial, you refuse to accept the truth that your food addiction is negatively affecting your life. You blind yourself to your addiction to protect yourself because it's scary to admit that you're out of control. It's also very embarrassing to confess that you're a food addict. People might suddenly picture you stuffing large quantities of food down your throat. You're also afraid that if you admit it, you may have to do something drastic about it. You might have to give up your favorite foods or say goodbye to the freedom of eating what you want when you want it. Remaining in denial, however, keeps you overweight and ruins your quality of life. As you complete the exercises in this chapter, you'll see this firsthand, but first take a minute now to reflect on the negative consequences of remaining in denial.

- **Denial feeds your addiction.** Instead of being conscious and aware of what you're doing and thinking, you put on blinders and ignore the problems your food addiction is causing. Your addiction now has room to grow and fester because you set no boundaries to contain it.

- **Denial stunts your emotional development.** Under your cool demeanor is a stuffed package of emotions longing to be expressed, understood, and acknowledged. The simple process of exposing these emotions diminishes the power of your addiction.

- **Denial is exhausting.** You buy cakes and goodies for the family to enjoy, but you eat them up before they come home. Then you need to replace them fast or come up with a good story about why they're missing. Hiding candy wrappers, waiting for people to leave the room so you can eat alone, running out at night to buy your goodies—it's all exhausting. All this energy could be used for more rewarding pursuits.

- **Denial isolates you from others.** When you live a life of deception, you block others from getting to know the real you. You reach for food instead of reaching for closer relationships with others. You hide your needs rather than opening up and asking for help. You isolate yourself with your food because you don't want anyone to see you eating. You try to hide your addiction, but your sheer body size gives your secret away. Your shame distances you from others.

- **Denial prolongs your pain and postpones pleasure.** By pretending you don't have a food addiction, you postpone the healing process. Your pain multiplies as you become more and more engulfed in shame and guilt. Confronting your addiction is the first step away from pain and toward a happier future.

Self-Assessments 101

Breaking out of denial is the critical first step to recovery, so please take your time in completing the following self-assessments related to weight, food, body image, and psychosocial issues. All these questions are here for a reason. Before you can turn your life around, you must see the *need* to turn your life around.

Reflecting on your responses will help you to free yourself from denial. You will form conclusions about your life to date and be motivated to act on those conclusions to create a better future.

This section requires introspection and realistic self-perception. You're the expert on you, and you're in the driver's seat—only you can internalize the need for change and progress. The motivation for change comes from within you.

Jot your reflections and insights down in a notebook or the free downloadable workbook at www.lindiscourtney.com (on the coaching page, under "tools"). Your insights will awaken you to the need for change in your life and provide the spark for doing something about it.

Your Starting Point

What is the most you have ever weighed?

How much do you weigh now? (Make an estimate if you don't have a scale.)

What is the recommended <u>range</u> of weight for your height? (See the chart that follows.)

How much would you like to weigh at goal weight?

How many pounds must you lose to reach goal weight?

Healthy-Weight Chart [2]

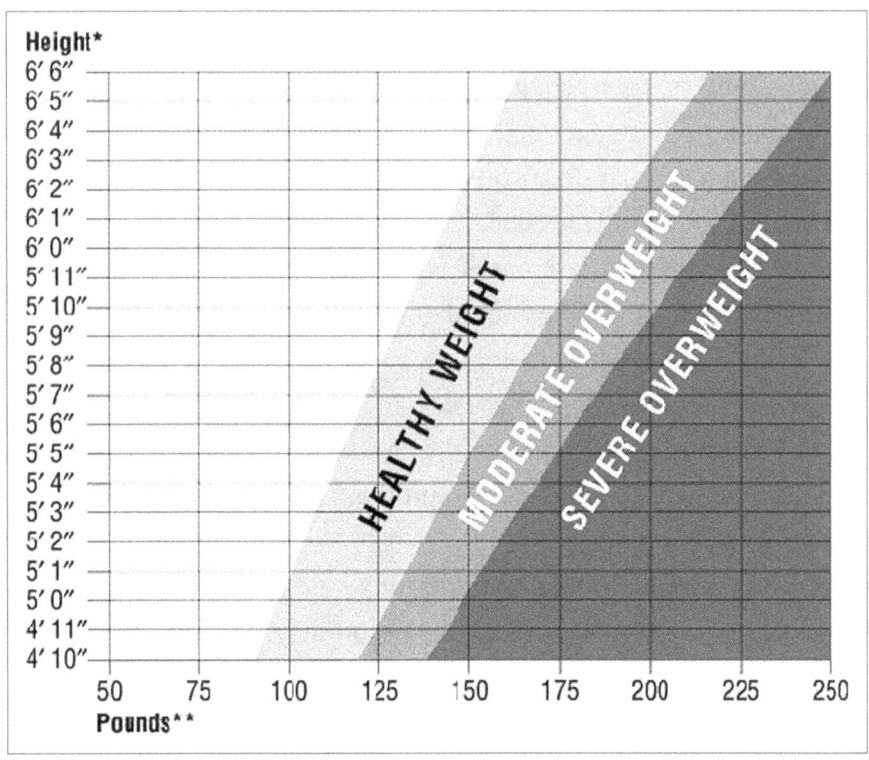

Your Weight Story

Do you ever wonder how you developed a food addiction and a weight problem? Plotting your weight story against a historical timeline gives you insight not only into when it began but also into the causes of the ups and downs that followed. Visualizing these "good" and "bad" periods on the timeline allows you to reflect on the times in your life when your weight and your life were in control and the times when your weight and your life were out of control. Plot your weight on the graphic that follows and do the corresponding exercise thoughtfully.

Age (in years)

Weight	15 yrs	20 yrs	25 yrs	30 yrs	35 yrs	40 yrs	45 yrs	50 yrs
240								
230								
220								
210								
200								
190								
180								
170								
160								
150								
140								
130								
120								

Weight (pounds)

Were there any major events that sparked a huge weight gain?

At what point in your life were you happiest? Did your weight reflect that happiness?

When were you unhappiest? Did your weight reflect that unhappiness?

At what points on the timeline did you feel as if you were most in control of your life?

Diets Don't Work

Many of my clients tell me that as soon as they announce they're going on a diet, they find themselves obsessing over chocolate and potato chips. We now know that the mere process of going on a diet can have serious negative effects, both physical and psychological. If you deprive yourself long enough, your metabolism starts to slow down and hang on to every calorie. You become cranky and hungry, and the scale barely goes down. If you stay on a low-calorie diet for too long, you become depressed or anxious. You can bear this for a little while, but at some point you crack and binge. You eat way more calories than you normally would, and you gain back all the weight you lost, and then some. Dieting is not a solution! It's the problem.

Take a few minutes to recall your personal experience with dieting:

How old were you when you went on your first diet?

Who or what prompted you to go on this first diet?

How many diets have you been on in your life?

Did you feel deprived and food-obsessed when you were on a diet?

Did you feel insanely hungry and binge afterward?

Have you ever been on a diet and kept the weight off for six months or more?

What is your overall feeling about "diets" now?

__ *Show me a good one and I'm on it.*

__ *I don't ever want to follow a strict eating regimen again.*

__ *No more diets, but show me a healthy food plan that satisfies me and I'd try it.*

Your Exercise History

You've probably heard about the benefits of regular exercise—faster metabolism, increased lean body mass, decreased level of fat, longer life, and more happy hormones. In addition, exercise can keep you feeling full for longer so that you naturally eat less. Despite all the benefits associated with exercise, most people avoid it.

For healthy adults, the Department of Health and Human Services recommends these minimum exercise guidelines[3]:

- 150 minutes (2½ to 5 hours) of *moderate-intensity* exercise (e.g., brisk walking) every week and strengthening activities that work all major muscle groups (legs, hips, back, abdomen, chest, shoulders, and arms), such as weight lifting or using your body's own resistance, two or more days a week

or

- 75 minutes (1 hour and 15 minutes) of *vigorous-intensity* aerobic activity (e.g., jogging or running) every week and strengthening activities that work all major muscle groups two or more days a week

or

- An equivalent mix of *moderate- and vigorous-intensity* aerobic activity and strengthening activities that work all major muscle groups two or more days a week.

Do you exercise according to the guidelines listed above? If no, why not?

Have you ever regularly exercised according to the guidelines? If so, when?

Which of these benefits of exercising do you like?
(If you think of more, add them.)

___ *Faster metabolism*
___ *Increased lean body mass*
___ *Decreased level of fat*
___ *Longer, healthier life*
___ *More happy hormones*
___ *Naturally decreased appetite*

Eating Patterns

Do you know you have an eating pattern? Perhaps you eat a certain way Monday through Friday because of structured activities like work or school. On the weekend, however, you may have a different eating pattern because you have more free time. We have lots of eating patterns if you think about it. You eat a certain way when you're on vacation, on Thanksgiving, and at parties. If you're overweight, you've engaged in a regular pattern of eating more food than your body needs. Are you aware of the specific eating patterns that have led to your weight gain?

How many meals do you typically eat in a day (breakfast-, lunch-, dinner-type meals)?

How many of these meals are typically healthy (not processed in a factory)?

How many snacks do you typically eat in a day (between meals)?

How many of these snacks are healthy (fruit, vegetables, dairy, grains, lean proteins)?

Do you engage in any of these food-addiction-type patterns?

- *eating more on the weekend than during the workweek*
- *continuing to eat even though you're full*
- *typically eating much faster than other people*
- *eating large amounts of food in one sitting*
- *going on eating binges for no apparent reason*
- *eating in secret*
- *eating to escape worries or trouble*
- *experiencing feelings of guilt and remorse after overeating*
- *intending to eat less but eating much more*

Do you have other concerns about your eating habits? Explain.

Calorie-Counting

Some people love counting calories and other people hate it. On the plus side, calorie-counting gives you a clear guideline as to whether you're eating the right amount of food for your body. On the downside, calorie-counting alone doesn't ensure that you eat the right kinds of food. Tracking calories for a variety of foods on a weekly basis is also a bit time-consuming. In a later chapter, we'll talk about a recommended food plan that focuses on portion size and healthy nutrition (instead of counting calories). Regardless of whether you like tracking calories, you know that it's scientifically important to your losing weight and keeping it off.

Do you know the number of calories a day you should consume based on your height and weight?

__ I track calories in my food. I eat about _____ calories a day.

__ I don't track calories. I guess I eat about _____ calories a day.

To get a good estimate of your recommended caloric intake, you can visit the U.S. Department of Agriculture's Supertracker at https://www.choosemyplate.gov/SuperTracker/default.aspx.

The Daily Caloric Consumption Chart[4]

Circle the number of calories a day you should be eating *if you want to maintain your current weight.* Then circle the number of calories a day you should eat *if you were at your target weight*.

Naturally, if you want to weigh ___ pounds, you would gradually eat fewer calories than you do now, moving toward the number of your goal weight.

Have you tracked calories in the past?

Do you see the value of being aware of calories?

Pounds You Weigh	Resting Calories *No activity*	Low Activity *2-3x times a week*	Moderate Activity *3-5 times a week*	High Activity *5-6 times a week*
100	1120	1450	1570	1680
110	1150	1490	1600	1720
120	1190	1550	1670	1780
130	1220	1580	1700	1830
140	1250	1630	1750	1880
150	1280	1660	1800	1920
160	1320	1720	1850	1980
170	1350	1750	1890	2000
180	1380	1790	1930	2070
190	1420	1850	1990	2100
200	1450	1880	2030	2180
210	1480	1950	2050	2200
220	1512	1970	2100	2270
230	1540	2000	2160	2300
240	1580	2050	2200	2400
250	1610	2090	2250	2410
260	1640	2130	2300	2460
270	1676	2170	2350	2500
280	1710	2220	2400	2560
290	1740	2260	2440	2600
300	1770	2480	2500	2660

Family Behavioral Patterns

Even if you'd like to believe you're completely independent of and unaffected by your family, you often inherit some of their habits, hurts and hang-ups. Comparing their issues with your own can be enlightening in regard to your understanding of your relationship with food. Numerous scientific studies confirm that people who experienced adverse childhoods (having been exposed to alcoholism, sexual abuse, or another type of trauma) have a higher tendency to become obese as adults. Food is often used as a nurturing or comforting mechanism to escape from past hurts. Letting go of food can be a real challenge, because it has been the solution to life's problems for a very long time.

Put an "x" next to any issue that you or any one of your family members has experienced at some point in his or her life.

Do you think your relationship with food has anything to do with your family's habits, hurts or hang-ups? Explain.

	You	Mother	Father	Sister	Brother	Grand Parent
Alcoholism						
Anorexia nervosa						
Bulimia nervosa						
Binge eating						
Compulsive thinking/ behaviors						
Depression/ anxiety						
Drug addiction/ abuse						
Emotional abuse						
Incest						
Mood swings						
Nightmares						
Phobias						
Physical abuse						
Psychotherapy						
Psychiatric hospitalization						
Rape						
Self-mutilation (e.g., cutting)						
Sexual abuse						
Stealing						
Other						

Your Body Image

Developing a positive body image and a healthy mental attitude is crucial to happiness and wellness. Unfortunately, most people don't think they measure up to what society calls beautiful. What do you think about your body? Does looking in the mirror cause you emotional pain? Take a moment to honestly respond to the statements below.

Check the statements that resonate as true for you:

__ *I think about how my body looks at least 10 times a day.*

__ *I tend to judge people by the shape/size of their body.*

__ *When I overeat a lot, I tend to isolate and avoid people because I feel fat.*

__ *When someone thin enters the room, I think about how and when I am going to diet.*

__ *I delay doing things until I am at the right weight.*

__ *I try to avoid mirrors. If I see myself, I get depressed.*

__ *I can determine whether it will be a good day or a bad day by what the scale says.*

__ *I constantly think about feeling or being overweight.*

__ *I feel self-conscious when I am with people who weigh less than I do.*

__ *I avoid eating certain foods in front of people because I don't want them to know what I eat.*

The Quality of Your Life

Do you believe you've missed out on certain aspects of a happy life because of your weight?

What has been the most upsetting and devastating aspect of being overweight?

What aspect of your life would be improved if you achieved goal weight?

Learn About the Problem

What Is Food Addiction?

Scientists have finally confirmed what those of us who suffer from compulsive overeating have known for quite some time: Chips, cookies, chocolate and other delicious fattening foods are addictive.

A study published in the journal *Nature Neuroscience*[5] studied three groups of lab rats for 40 days.

- One group was fed regular rat food.

- One group was fed bacon, sausage, cheesecake, frosting, and other fattening, high-calorie foods, but only for one hour each day.

- One group was allowed to pig out on the unhealthy foods for up to 23 hours a day.

The rats that were allowed to pig out became obese and their brains changed. They developed a tolerance to the junk food, needing to eat larger and larger amounts of it to get the same feeling of satisfaction.

The behavior of the rats clearly resembled drug addiction. Even after an electric shock was introduced, the rats kept eating the fatty foods!

What Are the Signs of Addiction?

The diagnostic criteria for substance dependence or addiction as noted in the Diagnostic and Statistical Manual of Mental Disorders (DSM-IV-TR) are:

- Substance is taken in larger amounts and for longer periods than intended.

- Persistent desire or repeated unsuccessful attempts to quit.

- Much time/activity is spent to obtain, use, or recover.

- Important social, occupational, or recreational activities given up or reduced.

- Use continues despite knowledge of adverse consequences.

- Tolerance (marked increase in amount; marked decrease in effect).

- Characteristic withdrawal symptoms; substance taken to relieve withdrawal.

Do You Have a Food Addiction?

Yale University researchers have developed a way to assess a person's dependence on food via the Yale Food Addiction Scale (YFAS).[6] Below are a few of the points on the scale that are used to determine whether a person has a food addiction.[7] Think about your eating habits of the past year and check the statements you can relate to:

__ I find that when I start eating certain foods, I end up eating much more than I had planned.

__ I eat to the point where I feel physically ill.

__ I spend a lot of time feeling sluggish or lethargic from overeating.

__ I find that when certain foods are not available, I will go out of my way to obtain them. (For example, I will drive to the store to buy certain foods even though other options are available to me at home.)

__ There have been times when I consumed certain foods so often or in such large quantities that I spent time dealing with negative feelings from overeating instead of working, spending time with my family or friends, or engaging in other important activities or recreational activities I enjoy.

__ I have found that I have an elevated desire or craving for certain foods when I cut down on them or stop eating them.

__ I have consumed certain foods to prevent anxiety, agitation, or other physical symptoms.

__ Over time, I have found that I need to eat more and more to get the feeling I want, such as positive emotions or increased pleasure.

__ I have had withdrawal symptoms when I cut down or stop eating certain foods. For example, I develop physical symptoms, feel agitated, or feel anxious.

__ My behavior with respect to food and eating causes me significant distress.

What do your answers tell you? Do you have a food addiction? Are you willing to write that down as a factual statement so that you can take the first step? I, _____, can honestly admit to having a food addiction.

What Causes a Food Addiction?

Based on the rat study and your own experience, you know that food addiction begins just like alcohol or drug addiction—through being overly exposed to the substance. Science backs up the theory, showing that industrial-processed food laden with sugar, fat, and salt—food that's made in a plant rather than grown on a plant—is biologically addictive.

How Do You Cure It?

Michael Pollan, author of *In Defense of Food*, proposes a not-so-original answer to the question of what we should do to combat food addiction: *"Eat food. Not too much. Mostly plants."* [8]

By reducing or eliminating your exposure to high-sugar, high-fat, calorie-rich, nutrient-poor, processed, fast, junk foods, you lose your desire for them. The food-plan recommendation I present in this book aims for healthy eating that satisfies you and eliminates cravings. Isn't that the ultimate goal, to be a naturally thin person who prefers healthy foods to unhealthy ones?

An important aspect of food-addiction treatment is learning new ways to cope with life's stressors and building a support team to listen and guide you in the process. Depending on your needs and the severity of your addiction, you may need a weight-loss coach or a counselor/therapist to help you work through the obstacles on the way to your goal.

Weigh the Risks and Rewards

Risks of Eating Unhealthily

Eating unhealthily is life-threatening. "Populations that eat a so-called *Western diet*—generally defined as a diet consisting of lots of processed foods and meat, lots of added fat and sugar, lots of refined grains, lots of everything except vegetables, fruits, and whole grains—invariably suffer from high rates of the so-called Western diseases: obesity, Type 2 diabetes, cardiovascular disease and cancer." [9]

The good news is that people who get off this dangerous Western diet see dramatic improvements in their health. "In one analysis, a typical American population that departed even modestly from the Western diet (and lifestyle) could reduce its chances of getting coronary disease by 80%, its chances of Type 2 diabetes by 90%, and its chances of colon cancer by 70%." [10]

Costs of Overeating

You have already paid a price for your overeating, but you may not have acknowledged it yet. I'd like you to take a minute to write down the costs of being trapped in your food addiction.

In what ways has your food addiction affected your finances, your relationships, your goals, your self-esteem, your career, and your overall happiness? Give examples in each area.

Rewards of Eating Healthy

On the flip side, changing your eating can improve your life drastically. Below is a list of the rewards of eating healthily.

Check those that you agree with, and add your own.

__ *I will look better and be more attractive.*

__ *I will feel like I have mastery/control over my life.*

__ *I will be able to shop for clothes in smaller sizes.*

__ *I will have a strong feeling of accomplishment.*

__ *I will be more confident.*

__ *I will have more energy for family and work.*

__ *I will be more positive and friendly.*

__ *I will take more risks in my career.*

__ *My health will be better.*

__ *I will be stronger, mentally and physically.*

Pros-and-Cons Analysis

There are advantages to changing, but there are also costs. List the pros and cons of changing:

Pros: What would be positive about changing?
Cons: What would be negative about changing?

Do you have more pros than cons? I hope so, because then you're ready to move on to the next phase.

Focus on the
Positive Outcomes of Change

"What the mind of man can conceive and believe, it can achieve."
—Napoleon Hill

Visualize Your New Life in Your New Body

Stephen Covey said, "All things are created twice. There's a mental or first creation, and a physical or second creation of all things. You have to make sure that the blueprint, the first creation, is really what you want, that you've thought everything through. Then you put it into bricks and mortar. Each day you go to the construction shed and pull out the blueprint to get your marching orders for the day. You begin with the end in mind.[11]"

The idea behind beginning with the end in mind is really about knowing your destination. Once you truly know where you're headed, it's easy to uncover the steps needed to get you there. If you visualize yourself having achieved the goal, you'll be more likely to believe it's attainable. Your mind believes you can do it because you *saw* yourself there. In fact, the more senses you use in the visualization process, the more likely you'll believe in your ability to attain it. "Human beings can alter their lives by altering their attitudes of mind," says author William James.

Studies of professional athletes around the world found that the best performers practiced some form of visualization. *The Gazette*, in Colorado Springs, Colo., reported that hours before scoring on a 71-yard catch against the Seattle Seahawks in 2006, Denver Broncos receiver Brandon Marshall had already visualized the play[12]. He planned what moves he'd make when he caught the ball, and he pictured himself breaking free from the defense. Marshall started using visualization as a boy when he daydreamed about football. "You go through what you're going to do and how you're going to handle different situations," he said.

I've used visualization quite successfully to prepare for job interviews. First, I would consider what might happen during the interview (i.e., what questions would arise), and then I would prepare my responses. I visualized myself having a good connection with the interviewer and projecting a confident and professional attitude. I also envisioned us laughing and smiling because the interview was going so well. Without fail, I'd go into the interview much more confident and positive than if I had skipped this process the night before.

Visualization works because 1) you anticipate what might happen by preparing and practicing and 2) you send a message to your brain that says, "Yes, I can do this. I know I can, because I just did it mentally, so I can certainly do it in real life." You show moving pictures to yourself to prove you can do it!

Everything we do in life is preceded by thought. We get to choose whether to use a positive thought that propels us toward our goal or a negative thought that impedes our progress. If you visualize yourself reaching goal weight and achieving your life purpose, you'll take steps to achieve it.

Take a few minutes to visualize yourself at your goal weight. What is the number on the scale? Where are you? What are you wearing? Are you inside or outside? What is the temperature? What do you smell? What are you thinking? How do you feel? Who is with you? What are you doing? The more senses you use, the more real your vision becomes to you.

*Write a description of your vision so you can review it regularly. At the bottom, in big bold letters, write, "I will weigh __."
Post this on your refrigerator or your morning mirror. Visualize yourself at goal weight several times throughout the day and*

before you fall asleep at night. Visualization is a common practice of champions who want to see their dreams become reality.

Your Moment of Truth

Are you ready to get out of the pre-contemplation stage? To do that, you have to dig deep and embrace rock bottom. Don't worry, you'll be quickly picked up again and eager to move on to the next phase. The point here is to get you to admit that you have a problem and that you don't want to have it anymore. **It's all about taking responsibility for the past, present and future.**

Please read this out loud:

I can quite clearly see that I am a food addict. I overeat even though I don't want to. I lose control around food. Even though I want to eat healthy foods, I have not been able to do that consistently. I don't like feeling out of control. This depresses me and affects my quality of life.

I weigh ___ pounds, but I want to weigh __ pounds. Based on my height and weight, I should be eating ___ calories a day. I'm eating way more than that every day. I don't exercise as much as experts recommend.

In the past, I thought that weight loss was out of my control, but now I see that my actions alone are 100 percent responsible for my current weight.

I want to be lean and healthy because the benefits far outweigh the costs. At this point, I don't know if change is possible for me, but I am certainly willing to contemplate changing!

STAGE

Contemplation

"Maybe I Will, Maybe I Won't"

CHARACTERISTICS OF CONTEMPLATION	HELPFUL STRATEGIES
• "Sitting on the fence" • Conflicting emotions • Not ready to change in the next 30 days	• Envision a brighter future • Identify barriers to change • Find more pros than cons • Create confidence in your ability to change

"There are risks and costs to action. But they are far less than the long-range risks of comfortable inaction."
—John F. Kennedy

Characteristics of Contemplation

Congratulations on admitting that you have a problem with food. You are now fully aware of what your food addiction is costing you in terms of time, energy and self-esteem. You're sick and tired of being overweight and being obsessed with body image. But as much as you want to be thin, you still doubt whether you can succeed. What are the costs? Will it be worth it? You've tried to lose weight a zillion times and failed. How will you be able to give up your favorites this time? What if you gain it all back? How can you believe this time will be different?

Don't worry, this chapter is jampacked with powerful positive brainwashing messages (okay, common sense) that will catapult you out of doubt and into belief. You'll learn how to channel your energy toward a greater purpose that's aligned with your life values. You'll see that you can express yourself through something more rewarding than food.

At the end of this chapter, you will examine *your* pros and cons of changing (and end up with a lot more "pros"). You will feel compelled to change. Instead of being in a dark cloud of uncertainty and hopelessness, you will become more solution- and future-oriented. You will be ready and willing to consider the possibility of change. You will begin to envision the possibility of a thinner you living a life of purpose!

Envision a Brighter Future

Do you have a purpose that guides your life? Do you have meaningful goals based on your personal values, unique passions and abilities? Does your life matter? Are you fulfilled? These are pretty hefty questions that you may not be able to fully answer just yet. That's okay, because this chapter is centered on helping you to discover your purpose, your values and your strengths.

This is critical to weight-loss success because having a purpose will keep your focus off food and on something much more exciting. Discovering what you want to do in this world, and why, will empower you to achieve much more than a lean figure. It will catapult you to your dream life, where you're actively contributing to others and making a difference in the world.

Rate Your Life

Before you discover your purpose and design your future life, you must take a good hard look at the major components of your life as it is today. Do you want to keep things the way they are (maintain the status quo) or make some significant changes? You typically can't improve one aspect of your life (reach goal weight) without getting help or resistance from the other parts.

I want you to look at the life you have today and compare it with the life you want. By doing this, you will be able to clearly see the gap between where you are and where you want to be. Acknowledging this gap is the first step toward closing it.

Please rank (0-10) each major life category below to reflect your current level of satisfaction in that particular area.

Major Categories	Rating (0-10) 0 = dissatisfied, 5 = a bit satisfied, 10 = totally satisfied.	What would make this area more satisfying?
Health & Fitness How do you feel about your level of health and fitness?		
Financial Prosperity Are you satisfied with your income and spending?		
Family Relationships Do you have close, warm, and friendly relations with your family members?		
Recreation Are you satisfied with the time and energy you put into hobbies, creative pursuits, etc.?		
Romance Are you in a loving, romantic, intimate relationship?		
Career Do you have a job you love that rewards your efforts?		
Contribution Do you believe that your life has meaning and purpose and that you contribute your skills to the world?		
Spirituality Do you believe in God and feel connected? Are you growing in wisdom, peace, love, and joy?		

Core Life Values

What do you value most in life? Family? Wealth? Personal accomplishment? These are examples of core values. Your core life values are values that you hold so deeply that they form the foundation for the way you live and move and breathe. They are the underlying force behind how you do your work, how you interact with others, and what strategies you use to get where you need to go in life. Your core values are practices you use (or wish you were using) every day in everything you do. Even though we don't always do what we wish we would do (such as eat right and exercise), the core values are there to guide us in that direction. True satisfaction is when you're living your life according to your core values.

In the next exercise, you will see 18 common core life values. Which of these do you share? Rank the top five from 1 to 5, with 1 being most important to you.

Rank

___ **Community** *To be deeply involved with a group that has a purpose beyond oneself. To perform in effective and caring teamwork.*

___ **Leadership** *To motivate and energize other people. To feel responsible for identifying and accomplishing needed group tasks.*

___ **Creativity** *To be innovative. To create new and better ways of doing things.*

___ **Personal Accomplishment** *To achieve significant goals. To be involved in undertakings I consider personally significant, whether or not they bring me recognition from others.*

___ **Enjoyment** *To enjoy my work. To have fun doing it.*

___ **Wisdom** *To grow in understanding of myself, my personal calling and life's real purpose. To grow in knowledge and practice my* religious beliefs. To discern and do the will of God and find lasting meaning in what I do.

___ **Expertness** To become a known and respected authority on what I do.

___ **Wealth** To earn a great deal of money (well beyond what's needed for my family's basic needs). To be financially independent.

___ **Family** To have quality time with my family members, to enjoy their company, and to contribute to their overall well-being.

___ **Service** To contribute to the well-being and satisfaction of others. To help people who need help and improve society.

___ **Friendship** To have close relationships with people I respect and have them respect me.

___ **Security** To have a steady income that fully meets my family's basic needs.

___ **Health** To be physically and mentally fit.

___ **Prestige** To be seen by others as successful. To become well known. To obtain recognition and status in my chosen field.

___ **Independence** To have freedom of thought and action. To be able to act in terms of my own schedule and priorities.

___ **Power** To have the authority to approve or disapprove of proposed courses of action. To make assignments and control allocation of people and resources.

___ **Integrity** To live and work in compliance with my moral standards. To be honest and acknowledge/stand up for my personal beliefs.

___ **Personal Development** To learn and perform challenging work that will help me grow and allow me to utilize my best talents and mature as a human being.

Do you live your life in alignment with your core values? How so?

In what ways do you live in conflict with your core values?

What would you have to change in order to live in alignment with your core values?

Discover Your Purpose

What does purpose have to do with weight loss? Everything! That's because discovering and embracing your life purpose is the No. 1 catalyst for living a joyful and passionate life. When your life is meaningful, you don't crawl into bed with a big bag of potato chips.

Your purpose, not food, becomes the engine that drives you, keeps your head cool through tough days, and gives you a true sense of meaning. You're more likely to hop out of bed in the morning before the alarm rings, excited about the day ahead. You know what you have to do and you're brimming with new and creative ideas for getting it done. Your inspired actions drive you closer to your goals each day.

I believe that you have been created for a unique purpose that only you can fulfill. This purpose will positively affect every aspect of your life—career, finances, family life, emotional and physical health. When you're in the zone and carrying out your purpose, you understand why you were born—how your unique talents, abilities, drives and passions fit into the greater plan—and you love your life. Your thoughts and actions are in sync with what you value. This level of enthusiasm is so vibrant that it will rub off on everyone you come into contact with. You'll radiate a renewed sense of confidence, power and passion. People will want to be around you, live like you, and help you with your mission. When you have purpose, you're participating in the greatest adventure of your life.

What's your calling?

Your true purpose is a "calling" that has been communicated to you in some form or fashion over the course of your life. This calling will most likely reflect your unique set of gifts, talents, abilities, passions, personality traits, and life experiences. It's quite possible that you have been given hints your whole life, but sometimes you're so wrapped up in living that you don't notice them. Once you do ultimately figure out your purpose, you will look back over the course of your life, and say, "It was so obvious! Why didn't I see all the signs and hints along the way?"

Discovery Time

Discovering your purpose is a critical first step in creating the blueprint for the next and best chapter in your life. Grab a pen and paper, answer the questions below and see what themes emerge. By the time you're done, your purpose should be so clear that a fire in your heart ignites. The adventure is about to begin. Dig deep, look within, and ask for divine guidance. Once you discover and pursue your purpose, your life will never be the same.

How would you describe your "perfect" life? Where are you? What are you doing? Who is with you? What are you doing work-wise? What are you doing recreation-wise?

Describe a "perfect" day where you can do exactly you want from the time you wake up until the time you go to bed.

What are you naturally curious about? What do you enjoy reading about, watching on TV, or learning about?

What would you like to change in the world? What about society makes you angry or gears you up for action every time you think about it?

What motivates and inspires you? Are there certain people, movies or places that give you energy and motivate you to think big or take action?

What do you do naturally well? Think about what you do well at work, at home, or in your free time. What do you think you're especially good at? In what areas and activities do you excel or shine?

What do you feel compelled to accomplish before you die? What are your life goals and dreams?

If you had unlimited time and resources and success was guaranteed, what would you do?

Name three role models (living or dead, famous or not, fictitious or real). What's special about them? What is it that you admire about each one?

Name three of your favorite books or movies. Why do you like them? What is the underlying theme? What aspects of the book/movie would you like to replicate in your life?

What legacy would you like to pass down to your children, grandchildren, etc.? At your funeral, what would you like them to say they learned from you?

What activities empower you and make you feel happy, productive and energized? This could be at work, at home or while participating in a recreational activity.

List five major accomplishments and why each was satisfying to you. Small or big, what made you proudest? This could be related to work, home, church, or recreational avenues.

Do you have a favorite quote, motto or verse? What is it? Why do you like it?

Brainstorm Your Purpose

I'm certain you uncovered some interesting information about yourself as you went through the exercises above. A theme has started to emerge revealing your innermost passions and abilities. This next step should reveal to you your life purpose.

Brainstorm: "What is my true purpose in life?"

Brainstorm freely now about whatever pops into your head as you consider the question "What is my true purpose in life?" Brainstorming means writing without censoring or questioning your thoughts. You don't even need full sentences. The key is to keep writing until you get to an answer that pierces right through you. Perhaps you'll laugh or cry, or maybe you'll have an "aha!" moment. Don't stop until you've discovered it. Use as much paper as you need.

Now create an elevator speech. Summarize your purpose in just a sentence or two, just as if you had only a few seconds in an elevator to share it with someone important.

My purpose in life is to ...

Sanity Check

Check whether your purpose passes the sanity check. If all the following statements are true for you, *score*!

__ My purpose is aligned with my core life values.

__ I can see how my talents, passions and abilities can be used to carry out this purpose.

__ Achieving my purpose will meet a human need (solve a problem, improve people's lives).

__ My purpose is inspiring, energizing and exciting to me.

__ My purpose is achievable in my lifetime.

__ My purpose is honorable. I am proud to tell others what it is.

__ I feel truly passionate about achieving this purpose (extra bonus points).

Working Backward

Once you know the ultimate destination and have visualized it, it's easy to devise the major steps that will get you there. Here's an example from my own life to give you an idea of what I'm asking you to do:

	Description of Tasks	**Completion Date**
10	I am a highly respected bestselling author of inspirational weight-loss books and a stay-at-home mom who has an abundance of time and energy to serve my family, my clients and the church.	Jan 2014
9	*Brainwash Yourself Thin* is a well-respected book that receives positive reviews on Amazon. It is moving up in the rankings.	Jan 2013
8	Publicity concerning the book's launch appears in newspapers, magazines, TV, radio, and social media arenas.	Dec 2012
7	Industry peers and experts in the personal-development field write positive reviews of the book.	Nov 2012
6	Electronic and paperback version ready for publishing for Amazon/Kindle.	Nov 2012
5	Marketing and PR plan is created and targeted audience defined.	Oct 2012
4	Website designed and functional in both English and Norwegian.	Sept 2012
3	Final draft edited and ready for production (English and Norwegian).	Sept 2012
2	Testimonials from readers, clients, and experts received.	Sept 2012
1	Final draft of book is professionally edited and designed.	August 2012

Write your road map from here to victory, starting from the place of victory and working backward.

Description of Tasks	Completion Date
10. Final Destination / Goal Realized:	
9.	
8.	
7.	
6.	
5.	
4.	
3.	
2.	
1.	

Naturally, each of the tasks above will have to be broken down into smaller tasks with shorter deadlines. But once you have the major steps, it's easy to define the minor ones.

Mental Rehearsal

You've already visualized yourself at goal weight, but now I want you to visualize yourself achieving your life purpose.

How has your life improved?

Whom do you help? Can you see the joy in their faces?

How have your finances improved?

How have your relationships improved?

What do you look like while carrying out your purpose?

Where are you?

Who's next to you?

What are you feeling?

What are you saying?

What response do you get?

Do this visualization exercise each evening before you go to sleep.

But What if You Don't Go for It?

If you don't follow through on your recovery from food addiction and don't realize your life purpose, what will happen to you?

What will the next 10 years of your life be like?

Whom will you let down?

What are the consequences of not changing?

What amazing things will you miss out on?

Are you willing to pay that price? Why not?

Identify Your Barriers to Change

False Rewards of Overeating

Every human behavior, including overeating, is goal-oriented. You do things for a reason. Subconsciously, you believe overeating actually helps you in life and serves a vital purpose. You believe food solves your problems or gives you a sense of control over your life.

This is one of the biggest reasons why you haven't changed yet! You live under the illusion that food supplies you with happiness, peace and security. On a conscious level, you know firsthand that it's not true. You have proof of the pain it has cost you in terms of lowered self-esteem and poor body image.

Tony Robbins, author of *Unlimited Power, Awaken the Giant Within* and the *Personal Power audio* series, teaches in his seminars that the biggest driving force in our life is our desire to meet our six basic human needs. Food addicts try to meet these needs with food, but you will learn to meet them by pursuing your purpose, growing in your faith, reveling in nurturing relationships, and embracing a healthy lifestyle.

Which of the six human needs below do you often try to fulfill with food?

Security/comfort

Do you turn to food for comfort when you feel insecure? The downside is that you later feel insecure because of your large body size and lack of control.

Uncertainty/variety

Do you try to get excitement and variety from chocolate, chips, fries, and candy? The downside is that this is not the variety of life that gives you real joy.

Significance

Do you experience a feeling of significance when you run out to the store for your favorite goodies after someone irritates you or doesn't behave like you want him to? Do you feel significant because you have money and the ability to buy your goodies whenever you need them? You might feel significant in the moment, but what you really crave is to be significant in the world.

Connection/Love

Do you cozy up on the couch in front of the TV with snacks when you feel lonely or unloved? Do you feel peace for a little while before you realize that you're still alone, and then you have to eat again?

Growth

You may think your goodies calm you down and keep you from screaming at the kids, your co-workers or your partner, but the only personal growth you really achieve is in your clothing size.

Contribution

Do you sometimes think you contribute to friends', family members' and co-workers' enjoyment by making and sharing your goodies? Does food connect you to others even though you don't always feel so connected to those around the table? This false sense of connection leaves you empty even when you're full.

Summarize your findings:

- *Which of the six human needs above is most important to you?*
- *Describe what foods you typically use to fulfill that most important need?*
- *Does the need get filled with food? If so, for how long?*

7 Beliefs That Sabotage Weight Loss

Have you ever heard of stinking thinking? It's when you engage in negative, counterproductive, self-sabotaging thinking that actually de-motivates you to the point of repetitive, consistent failure. Perhaps even as you read this book you think, "This will never work for me." Your negativity about your worth and capabilities is often the result of past programming from your childhood or another phase in your life. Get over it. It does you no good. Start with a new frame of thinking. If you don't throw away your negative blueprint, your body size won't change either.

Here are seven beliefs that sabotage weight loss.

"I can't do it, and even if I managed to do it, I'd gain it back anyway."

If you follow the *Brainwash Yourself Thin* healthy-eating guidelines and exercise regularly, you will be able to lose weight at a responsible pace while eating food you love. You won't gain the weight back if you adopt these changes for the long term.

"I'm doomed. Nothing works. I have bad genes. Something is wrong with me."

Your genes don't defy science. Healthy eating and exercise are the scientific way to reach goal weight and stay there. Certain foods hinder weight loss, while others accelerate it. When you follow the healthy-food guidelines in this book, your body will respond positively.

"I don't deserve it. I don't deserve to be attractive, thin, confident, and self-assured."

This sounds like programming from your past that needs to be discarded. If a good friend said she didn't deserve it, you'd quickly set her straight, wouldn't you? Set yourself straight now. You deserve it, just like everyone else. If you still don't think so, pull out a piece of paper and write down 10 reasons why you don't deserve it. I'm certain that piece of paper will remain blank.

"It's too hard. It's too painful. I can't stand being hungry or depriving myself."

Perhaps you've followed one or more diets in your life that were painful from start to finish. This time you'll be in control, creating a satisfying meal plan that gives you joy and strength. Once you start to eliminate trigger foods from your life, you are no longer a slave to them.

"I'll never be perfect and life will never be perfect, so why bother?"

Even though you may never have the body of a 19-year-old supermodel, you'll feel better if you're healthy and fit at any age. It's not black or white (a big mess vs. perfection). Set your goal to feel your best at this particular point in life.

"I need my food. It calms me, gives me control, reduces stress, and strengthens me."

This is the addict's perspective, that your substance is fulfilling your needs for happiness, peace and security. When you set meaningful goals in life and begin to achieve them, you will experience greater joy and meaning than any food can deliver. Let go of your substances and grab hold of life.

"I hate exercising. I'll never enjoy exercise, so I'll never keep it up."

Play with the notion that you are soon going to discover a type of exercise that gives you great joy. The definition of *joyful* is "feeling, expressing, or causing great pleasure and happiness." Doesn't that sound lovely? Imagine discovering a type of exercise you do regularly because you truly love it. It can enhance your vitality, your youthfulness, and your joy factor.

The Willpower Myth

The definition of *willpower* is "the ability to control oneself and determine one's action." If you're like most of my clients who struggle with their weight, you feel as if you come up a little short based on that definition. That's why I've created a new definition that's more attainable. Willpower is trying every behavior under the sun until it gives you the *result* you want. Willpower isn't some elusive character trait the lucky ones possess from birth that keeps them going back to the gym every day. Instead, it's an unrelenting drive to take regular and consistent action toward your goal. If you get stuck or sidetracked, you seek expert help (i.e., coaching) and keep working toward your goal until you achieve it. This is the way to the finish line; do whatever it takes.

Success in life rarely follows a straight line from start to finish. There are turns, setbacks, and roadblocks. Willpower is staying focused on your goal despite the interruptions.

The Feasibility Factor

At first I didn't believe I could ever lose 5 pounds, let alone 40, but I decided to try. I started to eat a bit healthier but held on to my favorite snacks in the evening. Then I started to walk to work instead of taking the bus. When I saw the scale go down week after week, I started to believe I could reach goal weight. I cut out more of my favorites, and surprisingly, I didn't miss them. Within five months, I lost 40 pounds, and I've kept it off. Looking back, it was a lot easier than I thought it would be.
—Susan C., San Francisco

The most critical factor of success is whether you believe reaching goal weight is desirable *and* feasible. If you don't think it is doable, you won't even try to achieve the body of your dreams. Do you believe reaching goal weight is feasible for you?

Of course it is! Let's take a look at the facts. You're overweight because you eat more calories than your body needs and you don't engage in enough exercise. All it takes to be lean and healthy is to eat less and exercise regularly so that you maintain a healthy metabolism, burn fat, and build muscle.

So, scientifically, weight loss is feasible for you. Your body isn't a freak of nature. You can lose weight by cutting calories and exercising consistently.

Of course, I realize that's easier said than done. You have a full-blown food addiction to deal with. How can you eat less and exercise more when your addiction seems to have a life and mind of its own? How can you turn down your favorite foods? Without your comfort food, how can you be calm and relaxed after a lousy day? Good questions. But I also have good answers. First, though, let me ask you:

- Have other addicts beaten their addictions?

- Have other overweight people developed healthy, lean bodies?

- Can people try on new behaviors that feel uncomfortable at first but ultimately fit like a glove?

The answer to all these questions is "yes." People who overcome their addiction experience mental enlightenment on a variety of levels. As you travel through the six stages of change, you will slowly form new ideas about yourself, your worth, your capabilities, and the ease with which you can incorporate small changes into your life. You will also come to the clear conclusion that letting go of your addiction *is* feasible.

Letting go of your food addiction is a process. You will actively try on a new strategy and adapt it to your style and personality. Every time you adapt to the new strategy, you will come closer to being free from your old patterns. Your belief in yourself and the process will strengthen.

Remember, even the wrong action is better than no action. Most people make many mistakes and experience relapses before they reach their final destinations. Learning by doing and gradually adapting to change is the key to success. You'll discover that you like your new routines better than your old ones, so the process of staying healthy becomes easier. If you follow the guidelines I propose in this book, you'll also see the number on the scale moving in the right direction. This can work for you!

Find More Pros Than Cons

Your No. 1 Reason

There are always pluses and minuses when it comes to making a major life change. Even though you truly want to reach goal weight and stay there, the enormity of the challenge before you might feel overwhelming. You may wonder whether change is worth it. Can you be successful at it?

Before you can determine whether changing is worth the time and effort involved, you must know why you want to change. What is your No. 1 reason for wanting to reach goal weight?

Experts say that having a compelling reason gives you a much better chance of achieving a major lifestyle change. That's because some days you may be tempted to give up or go off course. You might do well for a week or two, but then challenges arise. Stress, family and work demands disrupt your routines and test you. Someone hurts your feelings and makes you feel insecure. You might be at a party and everyone is eating your favorite cake. Having a compelling reason, ideally tied to your life purpose, should keep you focused and motivated.

I was compelled to reach goal weight because I desperately wanted to help others embrace their life purpose. If I continued to remain trapped within the confines of food addiction, I was of no use to the millions of people who needed a role model to guide them to freedom.

What is your No. 1 reason for wanting to achieve goal weight?

Write it on an index card and carry it with you in your purse or wallet. Read it out loud several times a day. It can be quite powerful.

The Journey May Be Better Than You Thought

In the next chapter, which focuses on preparation, I will share eating and exercising recommendations that can add joy and satisfaction to your life. My meal-plan recommendations involve foods that come from nature as opposed to a factory—lots of fruits, vegetables, lean proteins, low-fat dairy, and whole grains. At first you might find eating wholesome foods like this to be a negative thing but later discover that it's a fantastic thing. Healthy eating satisfies you nutritionally, so you don't crave junk food. It gives you energy and makes you feel emotionally stable. Combined with regular exercise, eating this way can dramatically improve the quality of your life. You can achieve the benefits of lean muscle mass, reduced appetite, fat loss, and a rise in happy hormones.

Mental Contrasting (Imagined Future vs. Current Reality)

Please think about your body for a moment and answer the following questions:

- *How do you feel about your current body's shape, strength, and flexibility?*

- *How do you see your future body, the one you'll have after you've incorporated joyful exercise and delicious healthy eating into your life? Describe that body and how you'll feel about it.*

Now, with that future body in mind, please answer *these* questions:

- *Is the idea of eating healthy foods and exercising regularly becoming more appealing?*

- *Can you close your eyes and see yourself as healthy and fit and enjoying the process?*

- *What are you doing? Who are you with?*

- *What is the expression on your face?*

- *Would you like to embrace this new and refreshing image and own it?*

Emphasize the Pros

Pros: *List as many positives about committing to change as you can think of. Consider how a healthier lifestyle will affect your confidence, your career, your relationships, your goals and your dreams.*

Cons: *List all the negative aspects of changing that concern you. Consider what you believe will be difficult about changing.*

Do you have way more pros than cons? Good!

Create Confidence in Your Ability to Change

Recognize Your Strengths

Do you have confidence in your ability to make positive changes in your life? People can and do change—it happens all the time. To embrace change, you must have self-confidence, faith in the process, and hope for the future. The opportunity to change is fully and readily available to you, but you must be receptive to it.

Fred, a 45-year-old accountant by day, secretly dreamed of starting a life-coaching business. He had completed his certification, but he was paralyzed by fear of taking the next step. What if he failed? What if he didn't get any clients? What if he didn't have the money to pay the bills? Instead of taking steps to launch the life-coaching business, Fred turned to food. He would graze on snacks throughout the day to distract him from his thoughts about the risks of starting out on his own. Within a year, Fred had gained 25 pounds and he was no closer to becoming a full-time life coach.

When Fred signed up for coaching, his goal was to move past his fears. I wanted to show Fred that starting and growing the business would not be a one-time event that either failed or succeeded. Instead, it was a process he could improve on every step of the way.

Fred was a successful accountant for over 20 years, so I asked him what he'd done to achieve that status.

"I just worked my tail off so the customer was always satisfied," he said.

I asked him how he'd done that.

"I would find out what the clients wanted and give it to them."

I asked him if he'd ever made a mistake.

He laughed. "Of course, all the time."

I asked what he'd do after making a mistake.

"I just admitted it and fixed it."

I had one final question for Fred. "Have you ever had to totally readjust your strategy to achieve the goal?"

"Oh, yeah, I'm always readjusting my strategy as new information arrives. That's life." We looked at each other and Fred smiled. "I get it. I already know how to make my life-coaching business successful."

The skills, resources, and experience that Fred had acquired over 20 years were the exact same elements he needed to launch and grow his coaching business.

Like starting and maintaining a business, losing weight and keeping it off is not a one-time event that you either succeed or fail at. It's a process. Even if you make a mistake now and then, it doesn't mean you failed. It just means you need to learn from it and make adjustments. Most likely you, like Fred, already have many of the skills and characteristics you need to ensure your success.

Recall Past Successes

There are millions of people who struggle with weight loss, but these same people are extremely successful in other areas of their lives, such as raising kids, running a business or leading others. Acknowledge your strengths, your past successes and the skills that got you there, because in most cases, these same skills will get you down to goal weight.

Name three things you are extremely proud of that you worked hard for:

1

2

3

What skills/personality traits did you exhibit that made these accomplishments happen?

1

2

3

What personality traits will help you to reach goal weight? (Are you motivated, goal-oriented, persistent, and flexible about new ideas?)

Do you have access to any special resources (books, classes, experts)?

Is there someone who will support you in your efforts (coach, friend, online community, family member)?

Do you have a special philosophy, belief system or set of values that will drive you forward?

Gear Up for Preparation

Finish the sentences below with positive declarations that express your feelings about your journey to this point.

I have an exciting purpose that I am interested in pursuing. My purpose is to …

After reading these first two chapters, I am much more confident in my ability to change because I know I have what it takes to …

So, the bottom line is that I'm no longer sitting on the fence. **I want to prepare for change!**

STAGE

Preparation:

"I Am Planning to Change"

CHARACTERISTICS OF PREPARATION	HELPFUL STRATEGIES
• Be ready to experiment with small changes	• Define your goals
• Collect info about changing	• Plan your eating strategy
• Plan to act within 1 month	• Plan your exercise strategy
	• Prepare for obstacles

"Before anything else, preparation is the key to success."
— Alexander Graham Bell

Characteristics of Preparation

If you're in the preparation stage, you're convinced that it's time to change. You're ready to collect information about what to do and experiment with small changes while designing your strategy. You've weighed the pros and cons of changing and have come to the conclusion that change is worth it. Bravo! The preparation stage puts you in control of the change process and sets you up for success. You will create goals and a preliminary plan of action and prepare for obstacles before they arise.

During this stage, you may have mixed emotions. You might be excited and nervous at the same time. That's good. It just means that you're fired up to achieve your goals. Don't be afraid, because when you create a good strategy and can predict and eliminate potential roadblocks, it makes the journey so much easier and stress-free.

Define Your Goals

Make Them SMART

The shortest distance between two points is a straight line. The plan you write in this chapter will give you a clear and direct path toward your goal and keep you from wandering or getting derailed. If you review and follow your plan on a daily basis, you will achieve it.

The first step is to create SMART goals—*SMART* for *specific, measurable, attainable, relevant* and *timely*. If your goal is vague, your outcome will be vague. A specific goal that is written down on a piece of paper has a much greater chance of being accomplished than a general goal in your head. That's because once it's in writing, it becomes more real, thought-out, strategic, and prioritized. You strengthen your commitment to the goal by writing it down. Only a tiny percentage of people write down their goals, even though research shows that when you do, you leapfrog over everyone else.

Breathe life into your goals by writing them down as we go through the exercises below. We'll challenge your goals so that you make them as SMART as possible.

But first, where is your starting position?

Current weight: _____

Healthy weight range: from _____ *to* _____ *pounds**

My target weight: _____

I am: ____ *overweight* ____ *obese (check one)* ____ *healthy*

---

*Check the healthy-weight-range table in Chapter One.

Now let's break it down into SMART goals.

Specific

I want to weigh _____ pounds.

I want to reach this goal weight because …

The benefits of reaching this goal weight are:

1.

2.

3.

4.

5.

Measurable

I will lose approximately _____ pounds a week. (Experts recommend 1 to 2 pounds a week).

Attainable

This goal is achievable. Other people have accomplished it, and I know I can do it because …

Realistic

This goal is something I am ready and willing to achieve. It is a realistic goal. I believe I can achieve this goal _____%.

Timely

I will achieve goal weight by _____ (month, year). This is a good time to achieve goal weight because …

Plan Your Eating Strategy

Ordered vs. Disordered Eating

At some point in your life, did you eat like a normal person: three predictable meals a day and perhaps a snack? I know I did. I remember being a kid, playing outside with my friends, and being annoyed when my mom called me in to eat dinner. I had better things to do. For the first 14 years of my life, I was not very interested in food. Eating was something grown-ups pushed me to do when I was either in the midst of something interesting or planning something interesting!

Of course, this changed drastically for me as an adult. Food went from being an inconvenience to being the center of my life. It was always on my mind. What about you? Has food taken center stage in your mind? The amount of time you spend ruminating about food is probably proportional to your weight. If you think about food a little bit, you're probably just a little bit overweight. If you think about food a lot, you're probably seriously overweight.

The solution is to stop thinking about food!

How? One way to dethrone food in your mind is to create a predictable structure regarding what and when you eat. Without such a structure, you might eat whatever comes your way *whenever* it comes your way and fuel your compulsion. If you always eat what you want when you want it, you may not have been truly hungry in years. You may not even know what real hunger feels like. Without a structured plan, you might spend a lot of your time, energy and focus on food. *What should I eat now? I really feel like eating chocolate. I know I shouldn't have that. Maybe I should have a sandwich instead. But that cake looks really good.*

By limiting your eating, you have time for a life in between meals. Many experts recommend six small meals a day to keep your metabolism running high, but if you have a food addiction, this can be dangerous. Eating too many times a day can keep your mind and mouth busy with food. Becky Lu Jackson, author of "Dieting: The Dry Drunk," writes "Random eating is the part of the disease that keeps us stuck in the feeding-frenzy energy—the eating compulsion/obsession." Overeaters Anonymous (OA), the 12-step program for overeaters, has a slogan, "Three meals a day, nothing in between, no matter what."

The opposite of ordered (planned) eating is disordered eating. Disordered eating is consuming more than your body needs for fuel; binging; and starving yourself one day and overstuffing yourself the next. Disordered eating can also include excess use of low-calorie foods or drinks to postpone or circumvent additional eating. Disordered eating is chronic and chaotic dieting. It's exhausting and it destroys your self-esteem.

If you want to overcome your food addiction, you must commit to ordered eating—creating a predictable structure of planned meals that fuel your body with nutritious foods. If you aren't physically active, you might plan three moderate-sized meals a day that are nutritionally satisfying. *Moderate-sized* means more than enough and less than not enough. It's a normal-sized plate of food for a person of your height, without second helpings.

If you engage in 30 or more minutes of exercise a day five days a week, perhaps you'll want to eat four healthy meals a day. Whatever you decide, the most important thing is that you follow a predictable structure of planned eating. By creating guidelines for healthy eating and following them regularly, you free up your time, your mind and your energy for other things in life. Instead of thinking about food, you're thinking about your fulfilling life.

Alcoholics have to abstain from only one ingredient: alcohol. You have to learn how to live with food in a controlled fashion so you won't be triggered to overeat compulsively. Your body will eventually get used to following a predictable pattern, and you will get used to planning your meals each day. It will become second nature, and with the right food plan, the weight will fall off.

What Type of Food Plan Is Right for You?

There's no one universal food plan that satisfies everyone's tastes, preferences and biological needs. You know what tastes good and satisfies you better than anyone else does, so you're going to create your eating plan with healthy foods you enjoy. I'll give you some guidelines and make some recommendations, but you will be in control. It's your life and it's your addiction-recovery plan, so you get to design your own food plan. It's easy to give up when you're following someone else's path; the way to become thin forever is to discover the way of eating that works for you. It should be something you truly enjoy!

The science behind guaranteed weight loss is eating nutritionally dense foods in the proper portion size according to your body's needs. Nutrient-dense foods have a high nutrient-to-calorie ratio, meaning they pack lots of nutrients per calorie. I'll present you with a recommended way of eating healthily that you can customize according to your needs. You'll be aware of calories but you won't be counting them. Instead, you'll track the number of items (portions) you have in a day.

The Goals of Your Food Plan

Here are the most important goals that should be achieved with your food plan:

- You enjoy low-calorie, highly nutritious meals and snacks that fully satisfy you and distribute nutrients throughout the day.

- You have enough variety in preparation, seasonings, ingredients, and taste that you're never bored with healthy eating. There's always something new to try and taste.

- You no longer experience cravings for unhealthy foods and are no longer tempted to eat between meals or binge.

- You can customize the meal plans according to your specific tastes and needs.

- You can follow your plan when eating at a restaurant or with friends and family

- You lose the pounds consistently, in a responsible manner, until you reach goal weight!

- You feel energized, strong, and satisfied, not deprived.

- You have a healthy, normal, stress-free relationship with food (which means an occasional non-healthy meal or dessert is okay in moderation).

The Building Blocks of Your Healthy Food Plan

If you're like me, your eyes glaze over when you hear about antioxidants, saturated fat, omega-3 fatty acids, and gluten. You just want to be told what you should eat to be healthy and thin for life. After decades of skyrocketing obesity rates resulting from overconsumption of processed foods, experts agree on this: Eat fruits, vegetables, proteins and grains. Perhaps you remember the USDA's Food Pyramid, which was around for decades. It received a lot of criticism because of its overemphasis on carbohydrates. Now the recommendations look like this.

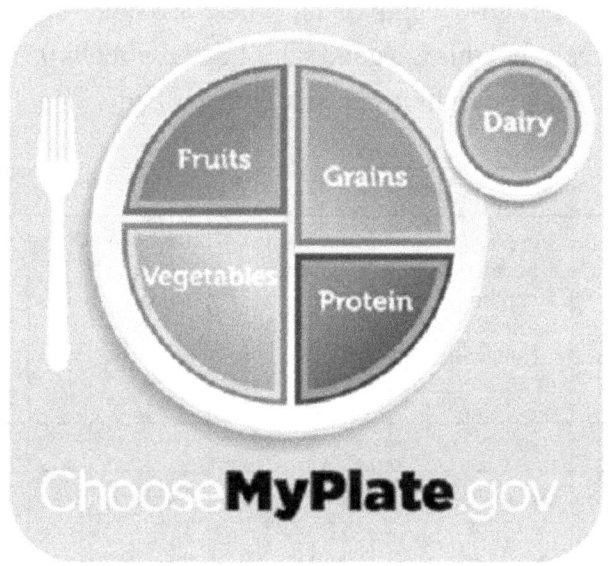

Source: USDA Center for Nutrition Policy and Promotion (CNPP)

The Brainwash Yourself Thin Recommended Daily Food Guide is aligned with the USDA's MyPlate recommendations. If you want to be forever thin, 95 percent of your meal choices should consist of fruits, vegetables, proteins, grains and dairy. Since there are good, better and best choices within each category, I've listed the best ones in the chart below.

Eating these healthy, non-processed foods will fuel your body and curb your desire to overeat or binge. When your body receives the nutrients it needs in the right amounts, your mouth, stomach, intestines, and liver will send messages to the brain that your energy requirements have been met. You will be satisfied after each meal. This is ultimate goal of the *Brainwash Yourself Thin* food plan, that you feel fulfilled by the food you eat and that you're relaxed around food. This is achieved when you let go of random eating and embrace planned eating.

This list is not all-encompassing. There are other healthy items that could fit in nicely, but this is a good start. Eat these foods 95 to 100 percent of the time to make weight loss easier for your body.

Fruits				
1 item 60 calories	1 apple 1 banana 1 cup fresh berries 1 cantaloupe	1 cup grapes 1/2 grapefruit 1 kiwi 1 lemon/lime	1 orange 1 papaya 1 pear ½ cup pineapple	1 plum 3 prunes 2 T raisins 1 cup watermelon
Vegetables				
1 item 1 cup (50 calories)	asparagus avocados beets bell peppers broccoli Brussels sprouts cabbage carrots	cauliflower celery collard greens cucumbers eggplant fennel garlic green beans	kale leeks mushrooms mustard greens olives onions romaine lettuce sea vegetables	spinach squash, summer squash, winter Swiss chard tomatoes turnip greens yams
Grains & Starches				
1 item 80–100 calories	1 slice whole-wheat bread ¾ whole-grain, high-fiber cold cereal ¾ cup oatmeal 1 whole-wheat tortilla	1/2 cup barley 1/2 cup brown rice 1/2 cup buckwheat 1/2 cup millet 1/2 cup oats 1/2 cup quinoa 1/2 cup rye 1/2 cup dried beans, lentils	1/2 cup peas (dried or green) 1/2 cup chickpeas, kidney beans, lima beans, miso, navy beans, pinto beans, soybeans ½ cup mashed potatoes	1 potato (6 oz.) 1 sweet potato (6 oz.) 1 yam ½ cup parsnips 1 ear of corn ½ cup corn (kernel) ½ cup green peas ½ cup whole-wheat pasta ½ ounce nuts/seeds

Protein				
1 item for women As shown (120-165 calories) **1 item for men** 6 oz. of protein (approx. 200 calories)	3 oz. beef, lean organic 4 oz. chicken 4 oz. lamb 4 oz. veal	4 oz. turkey 4 oz. venison 4 oz. cod 4 oz. halibut 4 oz. pork	3 oz. salmon 4 oz. sardines 4 oz. scallops 4 oz. shrimp 1 nonfat protein shake	4 oz. tuna 3 oz. lean meat 2 eggs 1 soy burger
Dairy				
1 item 90 calories	8 oz. buttermilk 8 oz. skim milk 8 oz. 1% milk	1 cup plain nonfat yogurt ¾ cup flavored yogurt 4 oz. tofu or tempeh	3 oz. nonfat cottage cheese 3 oz. nonfat ricotta cheese	1 oz. goat cheese 1 oz. low-fat Swiss cheese
Fat				
1 item 1 Tbs (90-120 calories)	Canola oil Olive oil	Coconut oil Sunflower oil	Flaxseed oil	Butter

What Should I Eat?

Below is a simple structure that can make planning meals easy. The amount refers to the number of items in a day based on the portion sizes in the previous table. Keep in mind that this is just a recommendation. Listening to your body is the most important factor for healthy weight loss. Check with your doctor as well so that you can devise a food plan that's best suited to you and your specific needs. For now, just notice the structure. It's straightforward, easy to carry out and predictable for you and your body.

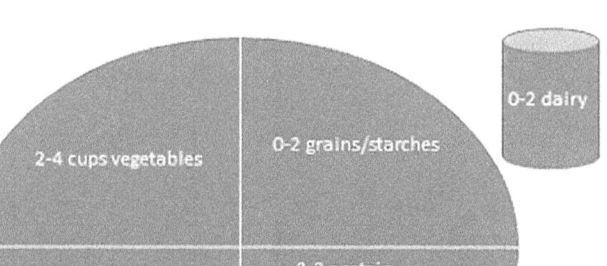

Brainwash Yourself Thin – What to Eat Everyday?

Two to Four Servings of Vegetables, Zero to Two Servings of Fruits

Eating two to four servings of vegetables and fruits a day will lower your blood pressure and help reduce the risk of heart disease, stroke, and probably some cancers. It's also great for weight loss because it meets your body's nutritional needs, making you feel more relaxed and satisfied. Your appetite will be reduced and your cravings limited or nonexistent. Limit fruit servings to two a day, because they're higher in sugar.

Two to Three Servings of Lean Proteins

Lean proteins such as chicken breast, eggs, tofu, veal, fish and shellfish are low in calories and provide high-quality protein with essential amino acids. Red meat is high in protein but also high in fat, so lean cuts are best. Avoid cold cuts (ham, turkey, salami, etc.) because they're loaded with preservatives. Non-animal sources of protein such as beans are good options as well because they're high in protein and low in fat. Protein aids in weight loss because you feel satisfied for longer.

Zero to Two Grains/Starches

There are good carbohydrates and there are bad ones. The good ones—whole beans, lentils, potatoes, sweet potatoes, brown rice, barley, amaranth, quinoa and oatmeal—are high in nutritional content, low in calories, and slow to digest. They keep you satisfied for longer, so you're not so concerned about your next meal. If you want an occasional slice of bread, tortilla, or plate of pasta, aim for the whole-wheat variety. These good carbs keep your blood sugar low, curb your appetite, and eliminate the need for snacking between meals.

I recommend the range of zero to two grains/starches a day because some days you may choose to have three protein meals with just vegetables. That's fine occasionally, as it will speed up weight loss, but you don't want to eliminate grains/starches completely. Combined with protein meals, grains/starches satisfy you and eliminate the temptation to overeat or binge. Find out what amount is best for you based on the feedback you get from your scale and how your body feels after each meal.

Zero to Two Dairy

Dairy foods such as milk, yogurt and cheese contain calcium, protein and carbohydrates. Choose fat-free or low-fat varieties. Eating dairy can reduce the risk of low bone mass in older age, and it provides essential nutrients, including potassium and vitamin D. Combining a dairy item like non-fat yogurt with blueberries is a delicious, healthy dessert.

I recommend the range of zero to two dairy items a day because you can get calcium, potassium, and vitamin D from non-dairy items as well. One cup of spinach, for example, provides 300 milligrams of calcium, the same as in a glass of milk.

One Fat

Our bodies need some fat every day. The good ones come from plants, nuts, eggs, lean grass-fed or free-range meats, seafood, cottage cheese, avocados, and certain oils (avocado oil, olive oil, coconut oil). It's also good to take one or two capsules of omega-3 fish oil a day, which is proven to increase metabolism and ward off depression.

Seasoning and Sauces

Make your meals tasty by experimenting with a variety of seasonings such as basil, black pepper, cayenne pepper, chili pepper, cilantro/coriander seeds, cinnamon, cloves, cumin seeds, dill, garlic, ginger, lemon juice mustard seeds, oregano, onion, parsley, peppermint, rosemary, sage, tarragon, thyme, and turmeric. You can enjoy low-calorie sauces and dressings such as soy sauce, oyster sauce, chile sauce, nonfat yogurt, Dijon mustard, salsa, tomato sauce, and balsamic vinegar.

What to Avoid or Limit?

Some foods should be avoided because they hinder weight loss, trigger binge eating or are just plain bad for you. Now that you're making a strong commitment to caring for yourself and your body's needs, try to avoid or limit the following items:

- **Soda (Diet and Non-Diet) and Alcohol**

Numerous studies have shown that people who drink diet soda gain more weight than those who don't.[13] Aspartame, an artificial sweetener found in diet soda, can raise your blood-sugar levels to the point where you actually crave unhealthy foods more. One study showed that the people who drank the most diet soda—at least two sodas a day—experienced waist-circumference increases that were 500 percent greater than those for people who didn't drink diet soda.

Furthermore, drinking diet soda throughout the day feeds the addictive process of putting stuff into your mouth for no nutritional reason. If you're thirsty, just drink water. Alcohol should also be limited or avoided. Alcohol and dieting typically don't mix well, because your body processes the alcohol first, leaving the carbs and fats to be stored as fat instead of fuel. Having a couple of glasses of wine can slow down weight loss—a 5-ounce glass has about 100 calories.

• Artificial Sweeteners

Despite popular belief, artificial sweeteners are not better than natural sugar if you're trying to lose weight. Artificial sweeteners can actually cause you to gain weight. Studies show that the more artificially sweetened foods and beverages you consume, the more you crave normal sugar-containing foods and beverages. That leads to overeating.

In one study, rats given food that contained artificial sweeteners ate more and gained more weight than those consuming natural sugar.[14] A separate study on 80,000 women showed that those who regularly used artificial sweeteners put on more weight per year than those who did not use them.[15] The consumption of artificial sweeteners can change your metabolism rate, insulin response and brain chemistry. Side effects include depression, insomnia, headaches, giddiness, loss of memory, nausea, and panic attacks. If you want to sweeten your oatmeal or cup of tea, choose natural sugar.

• Caffeine

Many people, me included, enjoy a cup of coffee in the morning, but consuming too much caffeine can cause you to gain weight. Caffeine raises the level of the stress hormone cortisol, which causes your heart rate and blood pressure to rise, which then stimulates your body to increase its stores of energy. This need for extra energy will cause your body to develop food cravings, most often for sweets.

• White Pasta, Rice and Bread

As mentioned earlier, there are good carbs and bad carbs. Good carbs are fiber-rich, natural foods such as fruits, vegetables, and legumes. Eating the bad carbs, refined and processed foods such as white bread, white rice, and white pasta, has been linked to weight gain.[16] Processed grains put a huge sugar load on the body while providing little nutrients. Replace these with the whole-wheat varieties.

• Nuts and Seeds

Nuts and seeds are great sources of protein, containing fiber, B-vitamins, calcium, minerals, and vitamin E. However, you must limit your use of nuts and seeds because they are extremely high in calories and saturated fat. And nuts can be too much of a temptation; most people can't have just one. Just a half-ounce of almonds has 80 calories, so you can occasionally sprinkle it on a yogurt or a salad, but measure the portion size so you don't sabotage your weight-loss plan.

• Junk Food

Nutrient-poor foods that are high in sugar and fat such as pastries, processed lunch meats and cheeses, ice cream, candy, cookies, cake, potato chips and corn chips should be avoided 95 percent of the time.

Have Your Cake and Eat It, Too

Since food addicts are often triggered to binge or overeat when exposed to junk food, many experts recommend 100 percent avoidance of foods high in fat, sugar, wheat, and flour. You know what's best for you. If eliminating these types of food serves you best, by all means keep them off your plan.

I wanted to have my cake and eat it, too, so I created the 95 percent rule. I eat healthily 95 percent of the time by choosing items off the recommended food list, but I allow myself 5 percent wiggle room. If I regularly eat six food items a day, that means I eat 42 items (6 x 7) a week, so if I want to follow the 95 percent-healthy rule, I can choose two unhealthy items a week (not *meals,* items). For instance, in one week I can enjoy popcorn at the movies and another day eat a delicious ice cream cone. This is what I call true recovery. You can have your favorites in moderation.

When you join forces with a weight-loss coach or other supportive partner, you can practice this so that it eventually becomes natural for you. To eliminate your desire to have more of a good thing, combine your 5 percent treat with a healthy meal. This eliminates the urge for more because your body is already satisfied with the nutrients it received from the healthy meal. As Groucho Marx once said, "Man does not live by bread alone. Every now and then he needs a cookie."

Portion Size: How Many Items a Day?

If you follow my recommendations, you'll eat five items a day at a minimum and 15 items at a maximum. What's right for you? That will depend on your weight, your activity level, and what items you choose to eat. Having four servings of vegetables in a day won't hinder your rate of weight loss, whereas eating two starches/grains a day might. Make adjustments based on what the scale tells you and, more important, how you feel after each meal. Are you satisfied? Do you no longer feel like overeating or binging? Good. Be sure you consume the recommended amount of vegetables and proteins every day.

How many meals will you have in a day? That's up to you. Some people choose to pack all their food items into three solid meals a day. Other people must eat more often for health or personal reasons. As long as you're having the right number of items a day, it doesn't matter how many meals you have.

Keep in mind that over time, the number of items you eat will gradually have to decrease to accommodate the needs of your shrinking body. You may lose weight quite successfully in the beginning by eating 10 items a day, but after a few weeks, you may have to go down to seven or eight items to maintain steady weight loss. You control the rate of your weight loss with the food choices you make and the number of items you consume.

Francis, a mother of five, reports that her weight loss was on track with eight items a day in the beginning stages, but by the time she got to her goal weight of 135, she was eating just five or six items a day. "Remarkably, just one item more than usual would send the scale in the wrong direction," she says, "so now I never go over six items."

Sample Weekly Plan: How to Track Your Weight, Food, and Number of Items a Day

I've created a sample seven-day food plan to give you an idea how easy it is to track your number of items. Naturally, you'll adjust the number of items based on your needs, your body's size, and your activity level.

Use this seven-day planner in your first week or create your own. Blank meal-plan forms can be downloaded from www.lindiscourtney. com (on the coaching page, under "tools"). Aim for variety in your meals from day to day so you never get bored with healthy eating.

Sample Weekly Eating Plan

DAY	AM Weight	Planned Meal #1	Planned Meal #2	Planned Meal #3	Snack	Veg. 2-4	Fruits 0-2	Protein 2-3	Grains/ Starches 0-2	Dairy 0-2	# items per meal 7-14	PM Weight (lbs.)
1	175	1 egg, 1 slice whole-wheat toast, ½ grapefruit	Baked salmon, 2 cups broccoli	Turkey breast, baked potato, cranberries	Nonfat protein shake	2	1	3	2	1	9	176
2	175	Breakfast wrap (turkey, vegetables, salsa, whole-wheat tortilla)	Grilled chicken with mixed vegetables in a whole-wheat pita	Top round steak with asparagus	Banana, apple	3	2	3	2	0	10	176
3	175	Oatmeal, 8 oz. 1% milk, banana	Turkey breast, grilled vegetables	Salmon, brown rice, salad	Berries	2	2	2	2	1	9	176
4	174	Low-fat yogurt, strawberries	Swordfish, black beans, tomatoes, onions, peppers	Chicken vegetable stir-fry with brown rice, oil	Melon	2	2	2	2	1	9	175
5	174	Low-fat cottage cheese with blueberries	Turkey burger on whole-wheat bun with lettuce and tomato	Grilled shrimp, green salad, whole-wheat pasta	Grapes	2	1	2	2	1	8	175
6	174	2-egg omelet with mixed vegetables	Shrimp, tossed green salad, .25-oz. nuts, raisins	Rosemary chicken with mushroom gravy, snap peas, yam	Kiwi	3	2	3	2	0	10	175
7	173	Oatmeal with blueberries	egg omelet with onions, peppers,	Chicken Vegetable soup		2	1	2	1	0	6	173

Weigh Yourself Every Day and Write It Down

You should track your morning and evening weight each day to remind yourself that this is a scientific process. What you eat directly affects the scale. Are you happy with the number you see? Does it reflect the good food choices you made, or do you need to make some changes? If you had three grains/starches yesterday, the number might have gone up. If you had zero grains/starches yesterday, the number may have done down. Did you eat eight items when you normally eat seven items, or did you eat 10 when you normally eat eight? Let the scale be your guide as you continue to make smart choices.

The Benefits of Drinking Water

Be sure to sip water throughout the day, about 8 to 10 glasses. Sometimes people mistake thirst for hunger. If you're well hydrated throughout the day, you won't have that problem. Before eating, ask yourself, "Am I truly hungry?" Part of the learning process is differentiating true hunger from emotional hunger. Later in this book, you'll learn re-patterning techniques for reprogramming yourself to do things other than eating when you're not biologically hungry.

Protein Shakes, the Easy Healthy Snack

If you exercise vigorously for 30 or more minutes a day (jogging, swimming), you might need to add an extra meal with protein and vegetables or add one or two nonfat, no-sugar protein drinks to your daily routine (midmorning and midafternoon). Protein-powder shakes provide a quick snack of high-quality protein without the fat and carbohydrates.

The three main protein powders are composed of whey, casein and/ or egg. Casein protein is good for weight loss because it's slow to digest and keeps you full and satisfied for longer. Visit a sports-nutrition center and tell them you're looking to lose weight and tone up. Make sure you read the labels so that you buy a protein drink that's nonfat and has no sugar. You don't want to have excessive calories in your midmorning or midafternoon meal. Buy a sample size so you can taste it before investing in a big container. Evaluate how your body feels before and after your workouts.

Fears About Changing Your Eating Style

How do you feel about changing your eating style? Does it feel a bit uncomfortable or downright scary? You've been eating a certain way for years, maybe decades. Perhaps you're used to having cold cereal for breakfast, a salami sandwich on white bread for lunch, and fast-food takeout for dinner. Trading all this in for vegetable stir-fries, grilled-chicken salads, and steamed fish will be an adjustment. Resistance is normal, but remind yourself that to change your body, you have to change your eating.

Sofie, a 35-year-old hairdresser from New York City, was adamantly opposed to eating vegetables. As a child, she hid her peas in a napkin or under a mound of mashed potatoes. Her memories of family dinnertime are filled with conflicts about eating disgusting foods. On the flip side, Sofie loved white bread, pasta and rice. She thought that anything brown would taste like poo.

To change her mind-set, I took her grocery shopping. In the frozen-foods section, I introduced her to more than 15 varieties of frozen vegetables. We grabbed a "Mexican fiesta" stir-fry (spiced tomatoes, peppers, mushrooms, carrots, onions and sweet chile), Vietnamese stir-fry (broccoli, baby corn, carrots, red peppers), and a Thai mixed-vegetable stir-fry (garlic scapes, Anaheim pepper, sweet peas, green onions, chopped, tomatoes). Then we bought a low-calorie cooking spray (only 10 calories a shot). In the seasonings aisle, we grabbed soy, teriyaki, and red-hot chile-pepper sauce. And to complete the expedition, we bought chicken-fillet strips, pre-portioned bags of brown rice, and whole-wheat pasta.

That evening we whipped up a "Mexican fiesta" chicken stir-fry with brown rice that rocked Sofie's world. She smiled at me between crunchy bites. "I had no idea this would be so good," she said. "I need a wok cookbook fast."

After our expedition, Sofie continued to shop like a pro. She lost over 14 pounds in seven weeks. "I'm a bona fide fan of vegetables," she said. "I feel so much more energized, and I actually look forward to eating them!"

If you have fears about changing your eating, know that change is possible. It's just a process. At first, you'll make the changes begrudgingly. You'll feel uncomfortable. After you do it a few times, however, you'll start to enjoy the new routine. It will become more comfortable. You'll notice the reading on the scale going down regularly, your clothes will get looser, and you'll have more energy. You'll start to enjoy the new way of eating and come to prefer it to the old way. You may even begin to crave your vegetables like Sofie does. Who knew that having a teriyaki stir-fry with just protein and vegetables could be so yummy? Who knew that having a cup of oatmeal for dinner could be incredibly satisfying? The uncomfortable becomes comfortable, and the comfortable becomes the preferred.

There's a science behind losing weight consistently and keeping it off for good. The people who are healthy and thin follow that science. Now you can, too.

How to Develop Naturally Thin Habits

Most of your life, you've heard behavioral weight-loss tips like "Eat sitting down" and "Put your fork down between bites." Perhaps you considered them mundane. I know I did. Now that you're highly motivated to change your lifestyle, you'll want to follow these tips to increase the likelihood that you'll get the weight off and keep it off:

- Plan your meals, ideally the night before, so you never get frantically hungry and make rash decisions.

- Weigh and measure food until you become an expert at recognizing portion sizes.

- Always eat sitting down. Food should always be on a plate. Never pick at food in the kitchen or anywhere else. Your meals should be relaxing affairs where you're aware of what and how much you eat.

- Make your meal last for 20 minutes by sipping water and putting the utensils down between bites. It takes 20 minutes for your brain to tell your stomach that you're full and satisfied.

- Try to limit or eliminate caffeine. It's an additive stimulant that can trigger you to eat more throughout the day. Choose water or green tea.

- Eat a variety of foods each week so you don't get bored.

- Keep a daily log of everything you eat and drink.

- Before visiting a restaurant, review the menu online so you can plan what you'll eat.

- Don't eat diet anything. Diet food is often loaded with fake sugars that set off the trigger to eat more food.

Plan Your Exercise Strategy

There are numerous ways of exercising, from joyful and fun to intense and vigorous. If you want to have a firm body and feel vibrant, you need to incorporate exercise into your life, period. Exercise increases your self-confidence and keeps you strong, both mentally and physically. It also affects the number of items you can eat in a day. Interestingly enough, it's easier to eat right when you exercise, because positive steps typically breed more positive steps. You're less likely to walk for 30 minutes and then come home and eat a pint of ice cream. People tend to reach for something healthy after a workout because they have a healthy mind-set.

Exercise Alone Won't Make You Skinny

As fantastic as exercise is, don't believe for a second that you can reach goal weight through exercise alone. One of the most widely accepted, commonly repeated assumptions in our culture is that if you exercise, you'll lose weight. This just isn't true. Millions of people exercise every week but are still overweight.

Perhaps you, too, have experienced the frustration that comes with sweating away at the gym for weeks on end and seeing no results on the scale (or in the mirror). That's probably why most people stop using their gym memberships a month or two after signing up. They just don't see the point.

Do you want to know why exercise often doesn't show results? It's because people think exercise alone is enough, so they don't change their eating. If you eat junk food (high-fat, high-sugar foods, including white bread, pasta, and rice), you won't reach goal weight. The most critical factor of becoming forever thin is that you eat highly nutritious foods 95 to 100 percent of the time.

Jennifer, a 30-year-old secretary in the oil business, came to me frustrated about her weight. Since she rode her bike back and forth to work each day, she couldn't understand why the scale wasn't cooperating. "I'm sweating up a storm every day with nothing to show for it. What's wrong with me?"

When I asked Jennifer what she typically ate in a given day, she replied, "I eat extremely healthy. A bowl of Cheerios, a sandwich for lunch, and a healthy dinner like grilled chicken, vegetables and rice for dinner." She was obviously pleased with herself.

When I asked her what she ate *after* dinner, there was a long pause, followed by a giggle. "I do snack in the evenings—who doesn't?—but the cycling should cancel that out."

When I asked her what she was snacking on at night, it was clear that cycling was *not* able to cancel it out. "Sometimes chocolate, or cookies or ice cream." Once she was able to cut out the night time snacking, the pounds started to come off quite easily.

If you eat the right amount of nutritionally dense foods, you will become thin with or without exercise. Adding exercise gives you incredible energy, top-notch health, and a body that's strong and lean. The best solution is to do three things: eat highly nutritious food and do cardio training and strength training. But if you can do only one of the three, eat highly nutritious foods because that alone can get you to goal weight.

The Benefits of Cardio

The benefits of doing cardio (aerobic exercise) several times a week are outstanding. Cardio includes any activities that cause your heart rate to increase. You know you're getting a good workout because you're sweating and your heart is pumping fast. Playing sports, jogging, swimming and walking are good examples of cardio exercises. Doing cardio on a daily basis can help stave off diseases like heart disease, osteoporosis, and diabetes. It will increase your levels of serotonin, so you'll feel happier and less depressed. Your self-esteem and body image will improve along with the shape of your body. You'll also sleep better at night and wake up more refreshed.

The Benefits of Strength Training

Even though cardio seems to get more press, strength training is even better when it comes to increasing metabolism and reshaping your body. Strength training doesn't always mean weight lifting. It's the use of resistance to obtain increased body strength. Free weights, medicine balls, resistance bands, and even your own body can create the necessary resistance. Push-ups, pull-ups, chair dips, leg lifts, jumping jacks, and stomach crunches are all strength-training exercises. There's also a host of DVDs with specific strength-training exercises you can do at home, guided by an expert.

Strength training helps you to create lean muscles, which increases your body's ability to burn fat, even for several hours after your workout. It also helps you to reshape your body. If you drop 25 pounds through healthy eating but *don't* strength-train, you'll be jiggling all over the place. You need to strength-train to tighten, firm, tone, and reshape your new body.

When and How to Start Your Exercise Program

So, when should you start your exercise program? For me, I couldn't even think about exercising for the first seven weeks. I just focused on following my food plan—that was enough of a challenge. After I dropped the first 15 pounds, I started to incorporate exercise into my life regularly. Even though I had a gym membership, I chose to order some highly intense, vigorous cardio/strength training DVDs that I could follow in my living room. So I basically went from nothing to high gear. You may decide to start slow, engaging in joyful exercise before working your way up to more intense routines. Let's explore both options.

Joyful Exercise

Remember the definition of *joyful*? It's "feeling, expressing, or causing great pleasure and happiness." How delightful. Imagine finding one or more types of exercise that give you great pleasure and happiness. It becomes something you do regularly because you truly love it. Stretching, moving and bending your body is a gift you give yourself. It increases your vitality, your youthfulness, and your joy factor.

I've thrown together a list of quotes from people who have discovered the joy of exercising. Feel their passion:

Exercise is my me time, and I savor it. … It's a mood-booster. … I love the endorphins and that I finish a hard workout feeling exhausted. … It wakes me up, makes me feel good and ready to start each day. … It gives me more energy, helps me sleep better, and makes me a less moody/cranky person. … It keeps me sane, healthy, confident, and challenged. … It makes me feel young and healthy and my day is never right if I don't exercise. … It relieves stress and makes me feel strong, attractive, healthy, and good about myself. … It always surprises me and gives me more energy than I thought it would. … It makes me feel amazing, mind and body.

Circle the exercises below that seem interesting to you:

Basketball, belly dancing, cycle cross, elliptical machine, gymnastics, handball, hang gliding, hiking, hip-hop/street dancing, ice skating, jet skiing, jumping rope, karate, kickboxing, martial arts, Masala Bhangra, parasailing, Pilates, rollerblading, rowing machine, running indoors, salsa dancing, self-defense, skateboarding, ski machine, skiing (downhill/cross country), snowboarding, soccer, StairMaster, strength training/weights, surfing, swimming, Tae Bo, tennis, treadmill, volleyball, walking outdoors, water aerobics, yoga, zumba

Which two excite you the most?

How would it make you feel if you were really good at these two exercises and saw the results on a slimmer, firmer you?

Could you commit to doing one of these exercises 30 minutes a day three to five days a week?

High-Intensity Interval Training (HIIT) Burns More Calories

If you're in pretty good physical shape and motivated to see results fast—in as little as eight to 12 weeks—you may be interested in learning about high-intensity interval training. HIIT routines encompass short bursts of maximum-intensity exercise separated by long intervals of low- to moderate-intensity exercise—e.g., running for one minute and then walking for two minutes.

HIIT burns more calories than just doing the exercise at a steady pace. That's because when you train at an intense level, your body can't supply oxygen at a fast enough rate to fuel the muscles. After the intense effort is completed, your body has to basically repay that "borrowed" energy by getting oxygen back to your muscles. The more energy your body borrowed during an intense effort, the more oxygen it owes (that's called oxygen debt). The larger the oxygen debt created by your workout, the longer it will take to repay it. This means that your body will burn calories for many hours after you've finished exercising. Nice.

You're a good candidate for HIIT if you're in good health, have no injuries, and are able to exercise for at least 20 minutes at a high-intensity level without exhausting yourself.

There are many approaches to HIIT, each involving different levels of intensity, lengths of time for each interval, and number of training sessions per week. HIIT programs may include walking, jogging, using an elliptical machine, a StairMaster, or a treadmill, or following aerobic/strength training routines on DVD or in a class at the gym. Choose a program that's not too physically demanding in the beginning so you can improve your stamina over time. You don't want to be injured the first week.

Perceived-Exertion Scale

On a scale from 1 to 10, your exertion level should be about a 7 during the high-intensity phase and a 4 during the low-intensity phases. A level 1 would be when you're sitting on the couch watching TV. A 2 might be standing, a 3 walking, and a 4 a brisk walk around the block. A 5 would be walking up a hill; your breathing is heavy, but you can still conduct a conversation. At levels 6 through 10, you're sweating, breathing heavily and not able to talk. A 10 is when you're giving everything you have to the task. As your conditioning improves over time, tasks you used to rate a 7 (walking uphill, for example) will become easy, so you'll have to start jogging uphill to keep yourself operating at a 7. That's the great thing about HIIT—you'll see a difference in your abilities and your body's shape.

Sample Jogging/Walking Interval Routine

Jogging one minute and then walking two minutes

Warm-up:	*Five minutes of walking*
High intensity:	*Jog for one minute at a level 7*
Recovery:	*Walk two minutes at a level 4*
Repeat:	*Do about eight cycles*
Warm-down:	*Five minutes of walking*

If you don't come down to a 4 during a recovery interval (you notice that you're still very out of breath and your heart is pumping fast), you may need to extend your recovery period or decrease the intensity of your jog during the high period. If the workout feels too easy, you can push yourself during the high-intensity part by running instead of jogging. You need to determine what's best for you.

If you'd rather take a more scientific approach, you can use a heart-rate monitor to evaluate your level of effort. When you're at the most stressful point in the workout (a level 7, for example), measure your heart rate. That's your maximum-intensity heart rate. During the recovery-interval periods (level 4), your heart rate should go down to 70 percent of your maximum-intensity rate. If it doesn't, you know you need to reduce the intensity of your workout or lengthen your recovery periods.

HIIT for Swimmers

If walking and jogging sound difficult, perhaps you want to test the waters of HIIT with swimming. It's less likely to cause injuries or put excessive stress on your body. Interval training with swimming is efficient in increasing your speed and endurance and burning calories.

To create your program, decide how many laps you'll swim in high-intensity mode and recovery mode. You may choose to swim freestyle at a level 7 for a lap, followed by the breast stroke at level 4 for two laps, before going back to freestyle again at a level 7. If that becomes too easy after a week or two, you can increase your level of intensity or the number of laps or decrease your recovery time. You can also drop the breast stroke and just focus on freestyle in both the high-intensity and recovery modes. When you're ready for an even greater challenge, you can incorporate the butterfly stoke into your routine.

HIIT in Your Living Room

If getting outdoors or to the gym is inconvenient, you may want to explore many of the fantastic HIIT programs available on DVD that you can do in your living room. A major benefit is that you don't have to create the program, watch the clock, or guess whether you're doing it right. You just do what the nice man or woman in the video tells you to do. Instructors tell you that if the workout is too difficult, you should march in place or take a break. In the appendix, I list video programs that have gotten rave reviews, some of which I've tried and enjoyed immensely.

Dig Deeper

> *"This is the first time that exercise is actually working for me. I started jogging and walking, and in just one month I've lost 10 pounds. I feel great."*
>
> **—Lauren, West Virginia**

> *"Interval training with swimming is very effective. Not only am I dropping pounds and building endurance, but I also get a very peaceful and relaxed feeling when I'm in the pool. This is my favorite exercise now."*
>
> **—Kathy, New York**

Whatever program you choose, the benefits are the same: You see improvements in your stamina within just a few weeks, and you notice that your body is getting leaner. As you progress, seek out more challenging exercises or increase your duration to avoid stagnation. You don't want to stay at the same level for long. The more you push yourself and increase the variety of your program, the more results you'll see in your stamina, endurance, and body strength.

I hope this chapter has convinced you that eight- to 12-week transformations can occur if you make serious changes in your nutritional intake and commit to an intensive cardio- and strength-training program. Forget about your past experiences—you *can* redesign your body.

> *After reading this section, do you have any new insights about exercise? Explain.*
>
> *What do you like about the concept of doing 30 minutes of joyful exercise?*
>
> *What do you see as the major benefits of doing HIIT when you're ready for advanced training?*
>
> *If you were to choose an exercise to do next week, what would it be?*

Sample Weekly Plan: How to Track Exercise

Most people don't plan to fail, they just fail to plan. This holds especially true when it comes to exercise. Instead of saying, "I really should exercise," you must write down what you will commit to doing in the first week.

To help you develop your strategy, I'll share with you the plan created by Laura, a lawyer in Maryland who decided she'd start out with a walk/jog HIIT exercise routine. Laura discovered an iPhone app that prompted her when to jog and when to walk. "I didn't need to think," she says.

At first she barely managed the two-minute jog, but within a month, she was jogging and walking for 30 minutes quite easily. Laura saw that her efforts paid off. "My body dropped two sizes in a month," she says. Now she's planning to run a 10K.

In the sample planner below, you'll see that Laura chose to do HIIT four days a week. Her planned level of intensity was a 7 effort when jogging and a 4 in the recovery phase when walking.

Day & time of day	Planned exercise	Planned level of intensity 4 – 10	Actual level of intensity 4 – 10	Joy factor (How you felt afterward) 1- not happy 2- normal 3- very happy	What will you do better next time? Extend the time, exert more effort, enjoy the process, or switch activities
Mon 9 a.m.	Walk & jog for 30 minutes of interval training (2 minutes jog, 2 minutes walk)	4 on the walk 7 on the jog	4 on the walk 5 on the jog	1	Enjoy the process
	break				
Wed 9 a.m.	Walk & jog for 30 minutes of interval training (2 minutes jog, 2 minutes walk)	4 on the walk 7 on the jog	4 on the walk 5 on the jog	2	Enjoy the process
	break				
Fri 9 a.m.	Walk & jog for 30 minutes of interval training (2 minutes jog, 2 minutes walk)	4 on the walk 7 on the jog	5 on the walk 6 on the jog	3	Exert more effort
	break				
Sun 9 a.m.	Walk & jog for 30 minutes of interval training (2 minutes jog, 2 minutes walk)	4 on the walk 7 on the jog	5 on the walk 8 on the jog	3	Extend the time (next week)

If she did what she'd planned, she'd note that under "Actual level of intensity." This way she could see, over the course of a week, whether she was living up to her expectations and working out at the necessary high-intensity level. She also recorded her "joy factor" after the exercise was over (not happy, normal, very happy). This reminds her how great she felt after exercise and increases her desire to exercise the next time. The last column is for self-reflection, allowing her to consider what she could do better next time.

Overcoming Obstacles to Exercise

The No. 1 reason people don't exercise is because they don't feel like it. The way to overcome this obstacle is to make exercise mandatory. When you have a job, you go to work even if you don't feel like it. People who are fit incorporate a routine and stick to it. They don't have to battle themselves in their thought world to get themselves to the gym. They've developed the habit of regular exercise and they just do it.

Studies have shown that people who exercise in the morning are more consistent with their exercise programs than those who try to fit it in later in the day. As you can guess, scheduling it later in the day allows the possibility for other, more urgent priorities to take its place. To overcome the I-don't-feel-like-it obstacle, try to wake up an hour earlier and do your exercise before the world disturbs you.

Spend some time to really think about when you'll exercise over the next week. The time you choose is as important as the actual exercise. Is it a time you can commit to regularly so that it becomes an ingrained habit?

Week #1 – Your Exercise Planner

Now is your chance to create your own exercise plan for your first week. It can be joyful exercise (no planned level of intensity) or some form of HIIT or a combination of both. Commit to what you will do this week, and write it in to the chart that you downloaded from www. lindiscourtney.com (on the coaching page, under "tools").

STAGE

Action:

"I'm Changing!"

CHARACTERISTICS OF ACTION	HELPFUL STRATEGIES
• Taking direct action toward achieving a goal • Practicing the new behavior for 3-6 months	• Transform your mind • Decide, commit and work your plan • Overcome obstacles • Create your support team • Reward yourself

"A journey of a thousand miles starts with one step."
—Lao Tzu

Characteristics of Action

If you're in the action stage, you're taking small steps toward achieving your goal weight. You're learning how to think differently so that you take the actions that give you the results you want. You're boldly venturing out and trying on new ways of eating and exercising. You have a plan that guides your steps, and you're keeping track of your progress and adapting your program accordingly.

The changes to your eating and exercise habits may at first feel a bit uncomfortable, but after a while the "uncomfortable" way suddenly becomes the comfortable way, and then it becomes the preferred way! Nothing succeeds like success. You'll get psyched up at seeing that your strategy actually works. The number on the scale goes down, your hope is restored, and your self-confidence and perseverance grow. You'll celebrate and reward yourself for the positive steps you take, and this will continuously refresh your commitment and belief in your abilities.

Transform Your Mind

Focus on What You Want

Your mind steers your life. If you think you can, you can. If you think you'll fail, you'll fail. Your thoughts determine your reality and define you. "For as he thinketh in his heart, so is he" (Proverbs 23:7).

The Law of Attraction, made popular by the best-selling book *The Secret*, simply says that you attract into your life whatever you give your focus, attention, or energy to, whether wanted or unwanted. What are you focusing on? If you focus on food, you'll eat it. If you focus on exercise, you'll exercise. Never, ever focus on what you don't want ("I'm so overweight"), because that's exactly what you'll get.

What do you want? If you want to be _____ pounds, devote your focus, attention, and energy toward that quest. What can you do to get there? When will you achieve it? How will you go about doing it? Your intentions and your actions get you there.

To achieve your goal, you will have to adapt new beliefs and thought habits befitting the thinner you. That's why the first section of the action phase is about controlling your mind. You'll have to practice letting go of your former way of thinking and replace it with a whole new thought process that will work to your advantage.

Write down what you want in life.

I want to weigh …

I want to accomplish …

I want to …

I want to feel …

I want to be …

I want to earn …

I can do it!

Take Control of Your Self-Talk

You talk to yourself all day long, and what you say affects your thoughts, feelings, decisions and results in life. If you think 46,000 thoughts a day and 95 percent are repeated from day to day, you need to control what you're saying to yourself. What will give you the best results, encouraging and motivating yourself or reprimanding and criticizing yourself?

Self-talk is powerful if you are positive, and it's destructive if you are negative. Remember that what you focus on expands. If you focus on the negative, you will attract negative developments in your life. If you focus on the positive, you will be motivated and equipped to succeed.

Listen in to your self-talk on a daily basis. Are these the thoughts of a champion? Are these thoughts going to help you achieve your goal? Is your focus, attention, and energy directed at achieving your goals?

Replace Sabotaging Thoughts

So, what do you do if you tune in to your thoughts and hear lots of negative statements like "I'll never achieve goal weight. It's too hard"? You must rebuke these lies by replacing them with positive (and more truthful) alternatives.

In the 1960s, psychologist Aaron Beck created a thought-tracking tool that was remarkably effective at curing his patients of depression and anxiety within just a few months. He simply taught his clients how to expose their negative internal chatter and swap them with healthier alternatives. While other psychologists were following the Freudian method of reaching into patients' past experiences, Beck discovered that the most powerful treatment was addressing patients' thought processes in the present.

If you regularly use the thought-changing tool below, you will be able to turn your negative thoughts into positive ones and move toward goal weight. Let me demonstrate this with an example. Imagine you were at your mother's house today and she offered you pizza, your favorite. You hadn't planned on eating pizza today, but before you knew it, you'd eaten three slices. On the way home, you beat yourself up with these automatic thoughts: "How could I? I've blown the whole week! If I can't say no to pizza, I'm never going to reach goal weight." Back at your apartment, you went directly to the refrigerator and grabbed a pint of ice cream. Your self-abasement continued: "Why not? I already blew the whole day, and it's not like I'm ever going to lose weight anyway." Watch how this scenario plays out in Beck's thought record:

The situation (the trigger)	Your feelings	Automatic thoughts	Case for	Case against	Alternative balanced thought	Re-rate moods
You ate the pizza at your mother's house (3 slices!)	Angry (50%) Sad (25%) Lonely (25%)	Why did I do this? I'm such an idiot! Why did I even go to Mom's? I should have known better. I'm such a failure. I have no one to help me.	I wasn't planning to eat the pizza and yet I ate it. I didn't follow my plan.	I'm in a learning process. I learned that pizza is a temptation and that it triggers me to overeat.	I made a mistake, but I can create a plan to avoid falling into such temptations in the future. I can also get a coach to talk to.	Hopeful (75%) Disappointed (25%)

I'm sure you don't normally say you're 50 percent angry, 25 percent sad, and 25 percent lonely. You think you have just one feeling, but learning to identify each of your feelings and breaking them down by percentages gives you much more information to work with. If you lump all your emotions into the "sad" category, you aren't aware that you're also "lonely," and knowing that you're lonely allows you to do something about it.

The tool encourages you to play the role of lawyers arguing for and against your case. Your automatic thought is that you're an idiot. In the case for, you support the statement by providing evidence as to why it may be true. In the case against, you provide information to discredit the assumption. And in the next column, you create an alternative balanced thought that's less painful and more truthful than the original thought of "I am an idiot." The balanced thought is a rational statement that looks at all the evidence and comes up with a kinder, gentler way of looking at the situation.

At the end of the thought-record process, you've come to feel 75 percent hopeful and just 25 percent disappointed. Though this was a fictitious scenario and actual results may vary, as they say, it's safe to assume you'll feel a good bit better for having gone through this process.

Avoid Common Thinking Traps

Beck noticed that his patients tended to fall into eight common thinking traps. See whether you're guilty of any of these, and then vow to create alternative balanced thoughts instead.

- **Catastrophizing.** This is extreme pessimism combined with the threat of doom. For example you might say, "I'm going to be overweight my entire life and no one will ever really love me." A more realistic alternative is, "I am overweight, but I am taking steps to lose the weight. I already have people who love me now, so I don't ever have to worry about that."

- **Generalization.** "No one loses weight and keeps it off for the long term. Everyone gains it back." Terms like *no one everyone, never*, and *always* are the buzzwords for generalization. Try to find exceptions to the rule. "Some people lose weight and keep it off. My Aunt Sandra lost 40 pounds and kept it off for five years."

- **Mind-reading.** "She thinks I'm fat. That's why she didn't smile when I said hello." You will never know what people are thinking. Even if you ask them, you won't know the truth. Give people the benefit of the doubt. If a person looks unfriendly, just remind yourself that something might be going wrong for her right now. It's not always about you. Don't try to read minds.

- **Polarized and rigid thinking.** It's black or white, right or wrong, good or bad. When Lulu eats food she perceives to be healthy, she says, "I was good today." If she has a café latte, she says, "I was bad today." She's also good at assessing a woman's size. "She's thin," she says of a petite woman. "She's fat," she says of the thin girl's companion. Looking at life through polarized and rigid glasses usually makes for a judgmental and critical person. This puts a lot pressure on yourself and those around you. Try to practice more flexible thinking that will deliver greater well-being.

- **Emotional reasoning.** This is when a person's emotions create her thoughts. "I feel so guilty. I ate the hot dog from the street vendor. There must be something seriously wrong with me." Janelle feels guilty after eating the hot dog, so her thought is that she must have done something wrong. Emotions aren't facts—they're just emotions. If you feel a strong emotion, consider the facts surrounding the feeling. In this case, the fact is that Janelle ate the hot dog, end of story. Maybe she was simply hungry. But whatever the case, next time she can pack a lunch so that if she wants to avoid hot dogs, she's prepared. No big deal.

- **Blaming.** "She made me eat it." "She invited me to an all-you-can-eat-buffet." "She said she baked it herself and I had to try it." "If I didn't have such an annoying husband, I wouldn't eat this much." Blaming others will keep you from goal weight because you avoid taking responsibility for your life. You can't control others, just yourself. Practice taking responsibility for your actions.

- **Filtering and magnifying.** Filtering is taking in the information that agrees with your preconceived notions and ignoring everything else. For example, Carol finds healthy foods boring and unsatisfying. At the mall, she sees a thin woman eating a tiny salad of lonely tomatoes and lettuce leaves. "I can never be thin," Carol thinks. "Healthy food is so boring." Meanwhile, the thin woman's companion sits across the table munching on a grilled-chicken salad overflowing with colorful vegetables, croutons, and pasta. Carol doesn't even see him. She's filtered him out. All she sees is proof that healthy foods are boring and unsatisfying. Magnifying is the opposite of filtering. It's blowing one piece of information out of proportion to support a preconceived notion. While walking around in the mall, Carol gets a glimpse of herself in the mirror. "I'm huge!" she thinks. "I'm bigger than anyone else here. I'm never going out again." If you fall into the filtering or magnifying trap, ascertain the facts and build a case for and against your theory.

- **Emotive language.** "I wouldn't be able to live with myself if I didn't reach goal weight within a year." Talking like this puts a lot more pressure on yourself. You've turned your weight goal into a life-or-death situation. Practice making less emotive word choices. Instead of the statement above, say, "I'll be really disappointed if I don't reach goal weight by the end of the year."

In the *Brainwash Yourself Thin Action Plan* that I will introduce shortly, you will learn how to track your negative thinking. Try to catch yourself engaging in any of the eight common thinking mistakes and then quickly turn the situation around by focusing on the facts.

Think With Positive Intention

Food is a drug that's available everywhere. You often feel as if you *have* to have some. You become obsessed with a certain food, be it tacos, burgers, pizza, muffins, or cookies. And giving in to the obsession is an addiction pattern that keeps you overweight.

Let's say you're at someone's house and there's a yummy chocolate layer cake on the table. You want it, you eat it, and hours later you regret it. In the heat of the moment, you needed it. You thought, "If I don't have it now, I'll explode! I deserve it! I have so much stress in my life."

This food-addiction thought pattern is the reason you keep the weight on. The secret is to expose the pattern and, once you understand it, break the pattern with new thoughts and actions. Your mission (with the help of a coach or other supportive person) is to become aware of the automatic responses to your triggers so you can replace them with new intentional conditioning that helps you stay in control and achieve your goals.

In any given hairy situation, you have many opportunities to impose new intentional conditioning to ensure a positive outcome. Let's say you're offered a cookie. Normally, if you're operating on automatic conditioning (as if you have no brain), you'll eat it. The model would look like this:

Trigger: You're offered a cookie
Action: Take it and bite into it

But since you do have a brain, and a very complex one at that, the actual process looks like this:

Trigger: You're offered a cookie

Thought: Yum! This will make me feel happy and soothe me.

Feeling: Desire for comfort

Decision: I'll take it!

Action: Take it and bite into it

Short-term result: You consume more food than you planned on and experience a feeling of hopelessness because if you can't resist the cookie, you'll never lose all the weight for good.

Long-term result: You weaken your ability to say no next time. You strengthen your food addiction.

Create New Mental Conditioning

How do you break out of the vicious circle of eating foods that derail your weight-loss goals? The solution is to create new mental conditioning that enables you to make smart choices automatically. Doing this takes practice. Most likely, you'll go through three phases before you fully master intentional thinking:

Phase 1: Somewhat Confident
(early stages of changing behavior)

Trigger:
You're offered a cookie

Thought (#1):
Oh no, that looks so yummy, I totally want it!

Thought (#2):

If I eat that, I strengthen my food addiction and hurt my progress. But it looks so good!

Thought (#3):

If I eat it, I'll feel terrible tonight and tomorrow morning when I step on the scale.

Thought (#4):

I'd rather feel good tomorrow and be proud of myself.

Feeling/emotion:

A little stress, but feeling confident, secure

Decision:

I'll say "no thanks."

Action:

Politely refuse the cookie

Short-term result:

Your self-confidence rises, and you've started to develop a new automatic response to triggers.

Long-term result:

You strengthen your ability to say no and really mean it.

Phase 2: Confident
(later stages of changing behavior)

Trigger:

You're offered a cookie

Thought (#1):

I don't want it. It will be too much sugar and not worth it.

Thought (#2):

I'd rather wait to enjoy my delicious wok dinner in an hour.

Feeling/emotion:

Peace

Decision:

I'll say "no thanks."

Action:

Politely refuse the cookie

Short-term result:

Your self-confidence rises further, and your new automatic response to this trigger has taken hold.

Long-term result:

You've solidified your ability to say no.

Phase 3: Totally Confident
(the new behavior is automatic)

Trigger:

You're offered a cookie

Action:

You say, "No thanks!"

True victory is this last phase, because the struggle is over. You don't care about the cookie anymore. Notice the thought process in all three scenarios—the stronger you become, the less time you spend battling yourself in your thought world.

Get What You Want in Life

You've now learned that your thoughts affect your emotions and your emotions affect your actions, which, of course, affect your results. But did you know that you can change any one of these elements (thoughts, emotions, actions, results) and get a different outcome? For example, if you're feeling depressed and force yourself to take a jog in the park anyway, the action of jogging could actually turn your depression into joy. You changed your emotion by changing an action. You can also change your action by changing your desired result. For example, if you want the result to be a weight of 135 pounds (when you currently weigh 170), you could devise a plan as follows:

Circumstance:
You weigh 170 and you want to weigh 135

Write down the result you want to achieve:

Result:
I reach 135 pounds in five months.

Ask yourself what action you have to take to achieve that result:

Action:
I eat no more than six items a day as part of highly nutritious meals. I write down what I eat. I hire a weight-loss coach and exercise for 30 minutes four days a week. I also train myself to think with positive intention.

Ask yourself what thoughts and feelings you have to have to take those amazing action steps consistently for five months:

Thought:
"I can definitely do this. I just have to treat it like a project!"

Feeling:
"I feel confident and empowered. I'm certain of my abilities."

The nice thing about intentional thinking is that you can start with any one element and it will change the others. You could have started with the thought "I can definitely do this. I just have to treat it like a project!" and built your strategy from there. Or you could have started with the feeling "I feel confident and empowered. I am certain of my abilities" and determined your outcome from there. Taking control of any one element changes all the other elements, and the result is a cohesive, positive effort. Rejoice! You have the power to change your life by taking control of your thoughts, emotions, actions and results.

Decide, Commit, and Work Your Plan

Congratulations on your decision to make positive changes in your life. By now, you have a rough idea of what you'll eat and how you'll exercise your first week. Success, however, lies in your ongoing daily habits. I've created a daily planner that will help you become mindfully aware of the new habits you're trying to adapt for a healthier and more energetic life. This is your action plan to victory, so own it. Set your goals and assess your progress daily. Challenge yourself to make small improvements each day.

Progress breeds more progress because you become more and more motivated as you get closer and closer to your goal weight. Any time you get stuck, you have two choices: Feed the addiction or feed the recovery!

The five-page *Brainwash Yourself Thin Action Plan* can be downloaded at www.lindiscourtney.com (on the bottom of the coaching page, under "tools"). After filling it out online, you can save it as a Microsoft Word document and update it daily. Open it now so you can follow along while I walk you through each element.

The Brainwash Yourself Thin Action Plan: Features and Benefits

Your Starting and Ending Points
(What is your goal and where are you now?)

Here you will list your start weight, goal weight, today's weight and total pounds lost to date. The purpose of tracking this on a daily basis is to remind you of where you are coming from and where you are headed.

No. 1 Reason
(Why are you doing this?)

Reviewing your No. 1 reason on a daily basis emphasizes the "why" behind the incredible changes you're making in your life. This is important to have in the back of your head when faced with temptation. Write down reasons that you would work hard to achieve.

Eating, Exercise and Weight Tracker
(Are you working your plan?)

On the second and third pages of the Action Plan is your weekly meal and exercise planner. Some of my clients plan their entire week in one sitting, while others like to plan one day at a time. Either way, review it each evening and make any necessary adjustments so that when you wake up, you're ready. These pages show you how your choices affect your weight loss.

Thought Mastery
(What should you think?)

To take the right actions, you must think with intention. This book is called *Brainwash Yourself Thin* because training your brain to think right on a daily basis is the critical driving force of your success.

The strategies below should be carried out daily.

- **Inspirational quote/verse/proverb:** Meditate on an inspirational quote, verse or proverb that motivates you to be strong and goal-oriented. You can pick a different one each day or focus on one a week. I like Napoleon Hill's "What the mind of man can conceive and believe, it can achieve" because it inspires me to believe in my vision. What positive beliefs do you want to embed into your head? Go and find them.

- **Morning monologue:** Reading a morning monologue each day can keep you to remain strong and firm against temptation. You might write something like this: "I am so excited because I am going to achieve my goal weight of ___ and my life purpose of _____. Every day I am getting closer to my goals. I love eating healthy meals and seeing the results of exercise. I can do this. I can weigh _____ and I can achieve my life purpose of _____." Read it several times a day and the I-can-do-it mentality will become ingrained in your entire being.

- **Thought tracking** (what thoughts should you replace with positive alternatives?):

  Use the thought-tracker to throw out any negative thinking that arises throughout the day. Practice changing the thought to a more balanced, truthful alternative. Over a period of days and weeks, you should notice that you are more prone to balanced thinking.

- **Intentional thinking** (*What thoughts will give you the results you want to achieve?*):

  Do you have a challenge coming up tomorrow? Plan for it by asking yourself, "What result do I want?" Then write down the thoughts, actions, and feelings that will give you that result. If you're going to a wedding buffet, you might want the result to be that you consume only four items (a protein, a vegetable, a drink, and a piece of cake). What do you need to think to make that happen? "Four items is more than enough to eat at a wedding. I can even enjoy the cake!"

- **Visualization exercise:**

  Each evening close your eyes and visualize yourself at goal weight and living out your purpose. Use all your senses to imagine what is happening around you. What do you look like? What are you wearing? What are you saying or doing? Who are you with? Who have you helped? What is the scenery? How do you feel? Revel in the joy of having achieved your goals.

- **Daily inventory** *(Did I do what I'd planned?)*:

  At the end of each day, you will ask yourself four questions: 1) Did I eat according to plan? 2) Did I exercise according to plan? 3) Did I purposely soak up inspirational messages (i.e., did you meditate on quotes/verses/proverbs and read your monologue)? 4) Did I think winner thoughts? Did I think thoughts that encouraged me to take positive actions?

- **Notes/journal reflections:**

  Here you can add your wins (what you're proud of), your challenges (situations where you didn't answer "yes" on your scorecard), and pinpoint focus areas for tomorrow.

Now that you know what to do with each element, fill out the forms to create your personal plan.

Overcome Obstacles

What to Do When Hunger Strikes

Be prepared for the fact that you may feel hungry between meals. You'll be eating less than you're used to, and your body will react by getting hungry. The sample meal plan for your first week is designed to load you up with highly nutritious, high-fiber calories so that you feel satisfied for longer. However, you may still feel hungry an hour or two before your next scheduled meal. Rather than eat ahead of schedule—you need to get used to waiting—engage in any of these activities. Feel free to add your own!

- *Do something you enjoy.* When I read, I forget everything. When I surf the web, I forget all about eating.

- *Talk to yourself and be rational.* "I can wait two hours. Food is available all across the country, in all the grocery stores, and in my refrigerator. It will all wait for me for the next two hours." If you use a little humor, maybe you'll see the fun in it.

- *Rate how uncomfortable the hunger is*, with 10 being unbearable and 1 being no problem at all. If you would rate having a tooth pulled a 10, your hunger is probably about a 3 in the grand scheme of things. That should calm you down, make you laugh, and allow you to go focus on doing something else.

- *Tell yourself* you're tackling hunger with the same nonchalance as a skinny person does. I can't tell you how many times I've sat in office meetings with skinny people whose stomachs were rumbling. Rumbling is normal!

- *Drink a couple of glasses of water.* People often confuse the sensation of thirst with hunger. Drinking water will satisfy you and possibly get your mind engaged with something other than food.

Whatever you do, don't have a meal two hours ahead of schedule, because you're teaching yourself that you can't wait when indeed you can, which you'll believe once you've done it often enough. Remember you're training your mind and body to eat at regular intervals throughout the day with large breaks in between (for the rest of your life!). After a few weeks, it becomes second nature. You'll even like the hunger feeling because you know you're losing weight and behaving like a skinny person. How cool is that?

Feel the Fear and Do It Anyway

Many of my clients admit that not eating when and what they want can be scary. When we talk about this in coaching, they admit to being perplexed. Rationally, they know that if they don't give in to a craving, they'll survive. They know that saying no to chocolate is no big deal, and yet for some reason it's a huge deal.

Do you also get nervous or feel highly uncomfortable when you don't get to eat what you want when you want it? Substances like heroin, cigarettes and food can be both physiologically and psychologically addictive. The more you use the substance, the more physiologically and psychological dependent on it you become. You may feel powerless without it if, deep down, you believe it provides security or comfort.

Your fear of not being able to get your substance can cause great anxiety. This might cause you to run out to the store at 11 at night to buy Ben & Jerry's Chocolate Fudge Brownie or rummage through the kitchen cabinets to graze on sugar cubes, chocolate frosting, or maple syrup.

There's a classic book, Susan Jeffers' *Feel the Fear and Do It Anyway*, that can advise us on handling this debilitating phenomenon. "At the bottom of every one of your fears is simply the fear that you can't handle whatever life may bring you," Jeffers says.[17] As a food addict, you're afraid that you won't be able to tackle life without your sugar fix. You must have it. You must have it now.

So, what do you do if you want to weigh ____ pounds and stay there? Can you continue to run out at 11 at night for Ben & Jerry's when the fear strikes? No. So how do you stop this pattern of craving followed by anxiety and ultimately submission? Feel the fear and do it anyway, Jeffers advises.

In this case, "do it anyway" means trusting yourself. Believe you can handle it. Believe the fear will pass. Most of the time, you give in to the fear too early and never give yourself proof that you can actually handle it. If you just feel the fear and let it pass, you'll know you can trust yourself next time. You can handle it. And each time you do, you'll trust your capabilities a little more. Nobody died. You survived and it was okay. After a while, you extend your boundaries. You conquered one fear, and you know you can conquer others.

"All you have to do to diminish your fear is to develop more trust in your ability to handle whatever comes your way,"[18] Jeffers says. Now, whenever I'm stressed about life and wanting my fix, I say to myself out loud, "Whatever comes my way, I can handle it." Try it and see if it empowers you too.

Tame Your Gremlin

There's another great classic out there, *Taming Your Gremlin: A Surprisingly Simple Method for Getting Out of Your Own Way*,[19] that can be applied toward tackling cravings and triggers. Let's take the same scenario: It's 11 p.m. and you're viciously craving chocolate and berating yourself. "Why can't I stop thinking about chocolate? What's wrong with me?" Instead of beating yourself up (that's your gremlin talking), just simply notice what's happening. Breathe. Notice. Listen to your inner dialogue; feel your body. Yes, you are craving sweets. Yes, you really would like to have them now. How interesting! Picture the phrase "I want something sweet" written in a fluffy cloud in the sky and just watch the cloud blow away. Watch it disappear into the distance and breathe. Simply notice that your mind and body wanted something sweet. Very interesting. Then play with your options. Do you choose to eat something sweet or do you choose to go to sleep? Do you choose to eat an apple and watch a late movie? You breathe, you simply notice your mind and body, and you choose the option that's best for you. There's no emergency. You have all the time in the world to simply notice. Breathe. Choose.

Adapt an Abundance Mentality (Not a Scarcity Mentality)

Do you have an abundance mentality or a scarcity mentality when it comes to food? One will keep you a slave to your addiction and the other will set you free. The abundance vs. scarcity mentality model, coined by author Stephen Covey, has been used in many fields, from economics to management to personal development. "Most people are deeply scripted in what I call the scarcity mentality," Covey writes. "They see life as having only so much, as though there was only one pie out there. And if someone were to get a big piece of the pie, it would mean less for everyone else."[20]

If you have the scarcity mentality with regard to food, you're often concerned that there won't be enough for you. You operate from a place of fear and control. You see slices of a pizza being passed around the dinner table and you think, "This can't be enough food to feed everyone." The fact that you eat a lot and quickly demonstrates that you have the scarcity mentality. "If I eat it fast, no one can take it away," you think subconsciously.

Another scarcity-mentality situation is when you continue to eat even though you know you're already extremely full. Imagine yourself all alone, enjoying a giant chocolate bar, eating it piece by piece, and feeling very full at the halfway point. The chocolate doesn't taste as good as it did when you started eating it 20 minutes ago. Now your chewing is labored, and your stomach feels sick. Why do you continue to eat it? Why don't you save the rest for another day? Because you have a scarcity mentality. You must eat it today or you know it will disappear.

Where does this scarcity mentality come from? Probably from your childhood. Perhaps your dessert intake was controlled or there was a limited amount of food in your house. You may not have had any control over what was served or when. Perhaps you were programmed to believe there won't be enough good food for you if and when you need it. Not having enough resources to survive is one of the basic human fears.

The best way to cure a scarcity mentality is to develop an abundance mentality. Covey writes in his book, *The Seven Habits of Highly Effective People:* "It is the paradigm that there is plenty out there and enough to spare for everybody."[21] One way to practice the abundance mentality is to tell yourself, "There is enough. In fact, there's more than enough to go around. There's food in the grocery stores, the gas stations and the convenience stores. Whenever I need food, I can get it. I can also save my leftover food for tomorrow and it will still be there."

You can also tell yourself, "Even though I didn't have much control over food when I was a child, now I'm an adult and I have access to food whenever and wherever I want. More than enough is always available. The world is overflowing with food, and I can have as much or as little as I want."

Practice this when you look at your plate of food, when you're waiting for your serving, and when you're halfway finished and full. You can always save leftovers for another day. If you want them tomorrow, you know they're there.

Reset Your Weight Blueprint

Did you know that most of us have a predetermined weight in our heads that we believe is our true baseline? Most of the people I work with have been at a weight plateau for at least six months. Have you plateaued at a weight that's higher than ideal? This number is your mentally acceptable baseline—your weight blueprint. You may not like this number, but it's yours and you've grown accustomed to it.

To start losing, you must mentally readjust that predetermined weight number or you'll sabotage yourself. If you weigh 175 pounds and your target goal is 135, you have to really believe you will someday soon be 135. Otherwise, if the number on the scale goes down to 159, you might be alarmed. Something won't feel right. Your mental weight thermostat was originally 175 and now suddenly you're at 159. You might panic. What's happening here? Even though you desperately want to be thin, you may be afraid of what being thin means. Will you suddenly be more vulnerable? Will you be weaker in a smaller frame, less able to tackle life's challenges or relationship stressors? Will people expect more from you if you're thin and attractive? Will you get more attention than you can handle? These types of concerns are normal.

Be a clever observer in this process. Notice how you react to the changing numbers on the scale. If you're pleased each time, fantastic. If you suddenly see a number and it scares you, just breathe, notice your fear, and then choose: Do I wish to continue with the program and reach goal weight? If you do, you'll have to reset your weight thermostat to a lower number. Anything above that is too high. Any movement toward it is good.

Create Your Support Team

Enlist a Weight-Loss Coach

Athletes need someone to inspire them, push their limits, and urge them across the finish line. CEOs of major corporations also have coaches to force them to think outside the box and push them toward greatness. What about you? Do you need a coach? Yes! Engaging a coach says you're worthy and have something of worth to give to others. It says you want to use your talents and abilities to achieve something great in this life.

It's close to impossible to achieve a major life change without a supportive person to inspire and encourage you along the way. "Two are better than one, because they have a good return for their labor: If either of them falls down, one can help the other up" (Ecclesiastes 4:9-10). Your coach is your collaborative partner. Even though you may have gotten excellent support in the past from a mentor, friend, or family member, a professional weight-loss coach has tools and strategies specifically designed to help you break through mental obstacles on the way to goal weight.

Your weight-loss coach inspires, listens, understands, encourages, and cheers you on. He or she is honest, respectful of your needs and as excited about your goal as you are. Your coach gives you honest feedback, uncovers your personal values, reinforces your inner strengths, ignites your passions and helps you pursue your goals boldly.

People who use coaches feel more encouraged, enthusiastic, and motivated to achieve the goal than if they were going at it alone. Some people need a coach to guide them in very detailed steps, whereas other people use a coach as a sounding board or as someone to hold them accountable.

Working With a Weight-Loss Coach

*"At first I was really skeptical about the whole
idea of weight-loss coaching, but then I found out
that it really worked. Yes, I learned to eat healthy and exercise,
but I also got so much more out of it. I even started to write a
book that had been floating around in my head for over three
years. I opened myself to dating and met a really nice man.
Coaching gave me permission to create the life I wanted."*
—Sharon, 31, New York.

If you and I were working together on a one-to-one basis, each week
we would do the following:

- **Create a plan for the week** (food and exercise strategy)

- **Develop structures and routines** that would best support your
  eating and exercise goals

- **Monitor your eating**. Did you eat according to the plan?
  Together we can strategize better ways to deal with certain
  situations, triggers or difficult emotions.

- **Practice intentional thinking** by writing down the results you
  want and the thoughts, feelings and actions that will get you
  there.

- **Follow the movement on the scale.** What should you eat
  today to give you the number you want to see tomorrow?
  What adjustments should be made to the meal plan? Are you
  expanding your repertoire of proteins, vegetables, fruits, grains,
  starches and dairy?

- **Acknowledge and address feelings.** What challenges have you dealt with this week? I'll help you acknowledge and address your feelings so you can meet these needs without food.

- **Review your exercise program, intensity level and length of workouts.** Are you enjoying exercise? Do you need to bring it up or down a notch? Is anything getting in your way?

Group Coaching

Group coaching is a good alternative to individual coaching because it costs less and many people are inspired by the group interactions. Most group weight-loss coaching programs are 8- to 12-week teleclasses delivered once a week for 60 minutes. Each week a new topic is presented and discussed. Some weight-loss coaching programs have forums in which participants can be in touch with each other outside of class, share recipes, and inspire each other with their success stories. See www.lindiscourtney. com for my group coaching class schedule.

Is Coaching Worth the Money?

Whether it's on an individual or group basis, weight-loss coaching is worth the money if the coach is an expert in the weight-loss field, has a strategy that works and knows how to get you to embrace a thinner mind-set. It will be much cheaper than buying diet books or diet products for the next 10 years!

Many people will argue that they don't have the extra money to pay for coaching. Can you cut down on grocery bills now that you're opting for a healthier lifestyle? Can you skip eating at restaurants and save a bundle there? Can you cut back on cable TV, movie tickets, or other leisurely pursuits that don't move you closer to your purpose? What price are you willing to pay to achieve goal weight and stay there forever? I'm sure it's way more than the cost of coaching.

The Advantage of Therapy

Sometimes weight is just one of the challenges you're facing. Hiring a therapist or other professional counselor can be the right decision if you have other things going on in your life that you want to work on, such as relationship, career, or financial issues.

If you had a dysfunctional childhood, the journey out of food addiction can be especially difficult. You may have spent a lifetime using food to cope with your feelings; you may have even needed the disease to protect you at some point in your life. But now that you're an adult, you have survived the traumas of your past. You are safe and you no longer need the disease to protect you. A major advantage of signing up with a therapist is that you create a strong foundation for your new life free from addiction.

Empower Yourself via 12 Steps

Research shows that when addicts help other addicts, it strengthens their own recovery. Beating an addiction is complicated. Even when you think you're free, nagging urges come knocking. Alcoholics, heroin addicts and food addicts are often said to be one drink, one shot, or one bite away from falling back into their diseases. Small relapses are normal, but going back full force into the black hole of addiction is an unnecessary tragedy.

Experts in the field of addiction have been incorporating a spiritual 12-step component into their programs for years because it's been proven to be effective at changing negative behaviors. Millions of people have recovered through them. The 12 steps are based on a spiritual growth process that begins with admitting that you are powerless over your addiction and a willingness to turn your life over to your higher power. Through the 12 guiding principles, you learn to examine your past mistakes, make amends, and live your life with a new code of behavior. Throughout your recovery, you help others who suffer from the same addictions.

Here are a few of the benefits of joining a 12-step recovery group:

- **You become honest and courageous.** Joining a group involves opening yourself up to others and letting them get to know the real you, with all your hurts and hang-ups. This can be daunting, but it makes you courageous. By sharing your story and your experiences, you can be an inspiration to others.

- **You meet people who are going through the same thing.** There's great comfort knowing that you're not alone and that others can relate to exactly what you're going through.

- **You get tips through other people's recovery.** You can ask other people in the group or a designated sponsor how to handle tough situations.

- **You discover that there's life without your substance.** The fact that others have recovered and found ways to live happy and exciting lives without their substance shows that you can also have a fulfilling life.

- **You're reminded of the consequences of overeating/binging.** Hearing the stories of others, especially newcomers in the early phases of their recovery, can have a profound effect on your own recovery. You remember the pain associated with being trapped in your food addiction. You're reminded of why you wanted to stop.

- **You have a safe place to go where you will not be judged.**
Finally, you feel like people understand you. Here's a place
where you can open up and verbalize the chaos in your head.
The others know what you're experiencing, so they won't
judge you. You feel safe, share more, and heal.

  John, a New York City security guard, was hesitant about
attending his first meeting. "I didn't know what to expect. I was
surprised to find a lot of really good people, with impressive
jobs and great senses of humor. When I listened to their stories,
I could totally relate. I kept coming back, practicing my three
planned meals a day. Within a year, I was at goal weight. My
battle with food was over."

- **You develop faith in your higher power,** which gives
you strength and hope during difficult times. Researchers
have discovered that 12-step groups are effective at beating
addictions for two primary reasons: 1) Participants replace
negative behaviors (overeating) with new positive routines like
attending meetings and reading positive literature, and 2) they
start to believe in something more powerful than themselves.
By developing faith in a higher power, participants are better
suited to tackle life's stressors without going back to their
addictive substance. I am a leader for a Celebrate Recovery
ministry in Norway and I can attest to the powerful influence it
has had on my life and those around me.

If you want to get more information about 12-step groups like
Overeaters Anonymous, Celebrate Recovery, and Food Addiction
Recovery, please see the resources page in the Appendix.

Join an Online Community to Catapult You Toward Your Purpose

Having an exciting life purpose to focus on will help keep your mind off food. Getting additional motivation and inspiration from online peers and experts can make the process more exciting. It may also help you to achieve your purpose goals faster and take them further than if you go at it alone. There are thousands of online communities to choose from. Whatever your interest, you can benefit greatly from connecting with others. Here are some reasons why being part of a community is invaluable:

1. **There's always something new**. Online communities can save you more time and energy than if you were on your own. With such a large number of people pitching in for the greater good, the information bank is overflowing. You'll have access to the collective brilliance of the members.

2. **Diversity**. Being exposed to people of different backgrounds, nationalities, economic classes, and personal preferences provides you with a diverse set of ideas and exposes you to an array of mind-sets. Your perspective on yourself, your situation, and your world might change. Coupled with diversity is the commonness of a group of people shooting for similar goals.

3. **Feedback**. Sharing opinions and getting feedback is priceless. An online community is a place where you can get answers to your questions and, in turn, share your experiences with others. You get support and offer support. It's also a lot of fun to celebrate your victories with others who have gone before you and others who will follow.

4. **Interaction**. In a community, you make time to interact with people who will motivate and inspire you to reach your goals. As humans, we need meaningful interactions with others, especially about the things that are foremost in our minds—our goals!

5. **Low cost.** The price of admission is either free or minimal. You get a ton of advice, tools, and interactions for much less time and effort than if you were to figure it all out on your own.

6. **Invitations to exciting events and other offers.** By being part of a community, you get invited to events that can increase your knowledge and expose you to new strategies. Free teleconferences are offered every month, hosted by experts who can provide an "aha" experience that serves as the turning point for your career or your health. If you want to join my community, please go to www.lindiscourtney. com.

Which of the support-team resources appeals to you most— weight-loss coaching, therapy, 12-step recovery, or an online support group?

What do you see as the advantages of joining forces with one or more of these people/groups?

Will you commit to trying out one of these opportunities this week? Which one(s)?

Reward Yourself

Acknowledge Your Successes

You should be proud of how far you've come in the process. You have a daily action plan that guides your steps. You're practicing new thoughts and behaviors that are becoming more comfortable. Give yourself credit in this early stage for taking the right actions. Heap compliments on yourself for attempting changes. Don't focus on what you did wrong; focus on what you did right. Use the abundance mentality to lavish yourself with praise, and back it up with rewards that excite you.

Below is a list of ways you can reward yourself for making positive changes to your eating and exercise routines. Check the ones you will use to acknowledge your successes.

__ *Announce your accomplishment to others and bask in the congratulatory remarks.*

__ *Book a session with a professional photographer.*

__ *Buy inspirational songs to upload to your mp3 player.*

__ *Treat yourself to a manicure or pedicure.*

__ *Buy some great-smelling lotion or perfume, buy a facial mask, etc.*

__ *Visit a creative place—a music store, a scrapbooking store, a bookstore, an art gallery.*

__ *Take a nap, sleep in, or just take a conscious break in the middle of the day.*

__ Watch an uplifting movie.

__ Take a day off—really off. Only do things you truly want to do.

__ Subscribe to a magazine that inspires you toward the life you want to live.

__ Give yourself a free pass to say no to something you wouldn't normally say no to.

__ Keep a wish list and buy one item every time you have a milestone to celebrate.

__ Get a massage.

__ Take a bubble bath.

__ Spend the day with a friend or family member you truly enjoy.

__ Make a reservation at a local hotel or bed-and-breakfast.

__ Give yourself a home spa treatment, with the husband and kids out of the house.

__ Buy yourself a new workout outfit or shoes or a piece of gym equipment.

__ Shop for a new outfit to fit your new body in progress.

__ Buy expensive healthy meals from time to time (sushi, gourmet takeout, lobster).

__ Go outside: Kayak, climb a rock wall, take a hike or lie by the pool.

__ Buy new pens and notebooks to journal your journey to goal weight.

__ *Buy yourself some free time (hire someone to help with housework or baby-sitting).*

__ *Fill your room, or your house, with fresh flowers.*

__ *Take a weekend trip to visit a friend you haven't seen in a while.*

__ *Get a makeover at a high-end makeup counter.*

Celebrate Your Learning Goals

It's one thing to reward pounds lost, but it's even better to celebrate the behavioral changes that will make the difference for years to come.

Check the learning goals you've achieved that you should be proud of:

__ *I am now satisfied with eating __ items a day.*

__ *I can eat a small dessert occasionally with my meal and I don't crave more.*

__ *I eat 20-minute meals so that I give my body time to feel full and satisfied.*

__ *I leave food on my plate because I am satisfied and no longer hungry.*

__ *I buy less, prepare less, serve less and eat less.*

__ *I don't panic if I'm hungry between meals. I know my next yummy meal is coming.*

__ *I have reduced my caffeine intake. This makes me feel calm and at peace.*

__ *I'm good at planning my meals and look forward to what I will weigh the next day.*

__ *My change in eating is something I can gladly continue for the rest of my life.*

STAGE

Maintenance (and Relapse):

"I Am Staying Strong"

CHARACTERISTICS OF MAINTENANCE (and RELAPSE)	HELPFUL STRATEGIES
Maintenance • Continuing commitment to sustaining the new behavior for 12 months or more • Avoiding temptation **Relapse** • Feelings of disappointment, failure and frustration • Learning and getting back on track	**Maintenance** • Create coping strategies to deal with temptations and obstacles • Plan for follow-up support • Reaffirm your goals and your commitment to change **Relapse** • Identify triggers that lead to relapse • Fight the relapse urge • Bounce back after relapse

"Success is getting up one more time than you fall down."
—Oliver Goldsmith

Characteristics of Maintenance (and Relapse)

If you're in the maintenance stage, you've let go of your destructive relationship with food and adopted healthy new eating habits. You have a lot more confidence in your ability to sustain this amazing change. The threat of returning to old patterns is less intense and less frequent. And if you continue to do what you did to get to goal weight, you will stay at goal weight.

The maintenance period lasts 12 months after the day you reach goal weight so that you're exposed to a year's worth of temptations (birthdays, holidays, vacations, weddings, funerals, job issues). Relapse can occur at any of the six stages of change, but it can be especially strong during the maintenance phase.

Relapse is normal (and not the end of the world), and bouncing back is fairly easy when you know what to expect. Don't be fooled into thinking that maintenance will be a walk in the park. Though you're motivated right now, be on guard! There are telltale signs that appear just before a relapse occurs and certain steps to follow to get back on track. Please take this chapter seriously because 90 percent of the people who lose weight gain it back. They never thought about or planned for the maintenance phase or for minor relapses. But you'll be prepared and armed.

Coping Strategies for Dealing With Temptations and Obstacles

Obstacles are a fact of life, but they shouldn't be feared. They should be welcomed. Obstacles are actually steppingstones. Think about the concept of an obstacle course. People actually go out and build a course that impedes progress! Why? Because the obstacle course draws out the best from the athlete. It forces the athlete to grow and develop so that he becomes more agile, flexible and strong. The course improves the performance of the athlete so that he's in a better position to compete in the future. Can it be that the obstacles in our life are also designed to improve our performance? Can it be that obstacles enable us to grow in ability and faith?

As Muhammad Ali, the famous American boxer, said, "The toughest opponent you'll ever face is yourself." We usually get in the way of our own success. And that means we also have the ability to get out of the way!

Whenever you're faced with a temptation or an obstacle, ask yourself, "Will my next action feed the disease or feed the recovery?" If you reach for the food item, you're feeding the disease. If you take new positive actions, you're feeding the recovery. Below are three positive ways to get past obstacles and temptations.

Countering

Countering is all about substituting healthy responses in exchange for unhealthy ones. Let's say you're thinking about eating a piece of chocolate cake at 5 p.m. (hmmm, why do all my examples have to do with chocolate?). Instead of going to the kitchen to eat the cake, you can counter that urge with an alternative action. The best action is one that will satisfy the positive intentions behind you wanting the chocolate cake.

Let's say you wanted it to feel relaxed—so go find an activity that will truly relax you (self-massage, listening to a deep-relaxation CD, watching a romantic film, etc.). Or perhaps you're looking to the chocolate cake for an escape from the lousy day you had. An appropriate activity for escapism might be renting a really good film or calling a friend. If you're sad and lonely and the cake was there to comfort you, perhaps you could join a community on the web, set up a profile, and reach out to others.

Countering activities are most effective when they achieve what you really want when you want it. Here's a list of ideas for addressing various emotions. Jot your ideas down next to mine.

Are You Restless, Bored?

- Call or visit a friend

- Read a book; read positive quotes and verses

- Exercise (go for a walk)

Are You Stressed, Anxious?

- Do deep-breathing exercises

- Listen to a relaxation audio

- Take a hot shower or bath

Are You Uncertain, Confused, Insecure?

- Journal your feelings

- Take strategy steps toward your purpose

- Brainstorm about solutions to concerns

- Call a trusted friend or family member

- Hire a coach, therapist, or sponsor

Depressed, Lonely, Hopeless

- Reach out to a friend; create a blog

- Go to sleep—the morning is always brighter

- Watch comedy

Anchoring

Anchors are your own personal cues and triggers to remind you of your goals and put you in touch with your self-drive and motivation. An anchor can come in any shape or size. It can be a particular outfit you wear to feel confident, a rabbit's foot in your pocket to remind you that you're lucky, or a perfume that inspires you to be powerful and strong.

Anchoring is a great tool for overcoming a temptation. Let's say you're about to raid the refrigerator but hanging on the refrigerator door is the picture of your dream home by the sea. The picture is an anchor to remind you that losing the weight is a major aspect of the overall career makeover that will ultimately enable you to get that house.

Take a minute and think about what situations bring out the greatest temptation for you, and then design an anchor to remind you to stay goal-focused in the presence of that temptation. You can use jewelry, music CDs, a relaxation session, index cards with quotes—be creative.

List difficult situations, locations or people that tempt you to overeat:

Come up with ideas for anchors that would keep you focused on your goals:

Re-patterning

Re-patterning is undoing the beliefs, behaviors and negative emotions that keep you in your food addiction. These addictive patterns or programming are so ingrained that it might be hard to adapt to new, healthier alternatives. To get rid of these sabotaging patterns, you have to become aware of them so they can be addressed.

For example, I had a pattern of eating after guests left my home after a party. I'd nibble as I cleaned up. I was successful at weight loss overall, but I'd get thrown off track whenever I had guests over. I needed to re-pattern myself. First I had to become aware and ask myself why I was nibbling after they left. Was I stressed out? Had I not enjoyed myself? Had I not eaten enough when my guests were here? What was it? Then I needed to ask myself how I could break the pattern.

The solution was that after friends and family left my home, I kindly asked my husband to clean up the kitchen, so that I could retreat to my room and reflect about the party in my journal. This was extremely useful re-patterning because I avoided the extra food and I set aside time to find out what was really bothering me. I discovered that whenever I have guests, I worry too much about what they think—about my house (was it clean enough?), about the tablecloth (had they seen the wrinkles?), about the food (did it taste good?). After journaling, I realized how ridiculous I was being. My guests had come to the party because they enjoy our company. After my "aha" experience, I chose to create a permanent pattern of retreating into my room after parties to avoid temptation.

Are there difficult situations, people, or events that prompt you to overeat? What are they?

What do you usually do in those situations (I.e., how and when do you overeat)?

What can you do differently next time? What new pattern can you create?

Recurring Thoughts

Sometimes you have something on your mind that just won't go away. It may concern an area of your life—career, weight, relationships, family, money—that you wish were different. Rather than trying to distract yourself from the problem by eating unhealthily, commit to solving the issue. Write down the key thoughts/themes and then write down how you would like this area to be improved. Once you've done that, you can prioritize your ideas and take action to address them in a positive way (without food!).

Complete the following:

There are one or more areas of my life that warrant my attention. They are ….

How do I want these areas to be improved?

Solving Challenges

It's been said that people use only 10 percent of their brain capacity. When a challenge or obstacle arises, sit down with a piece of paper and write the challenge on the top. Then brainstorm for 15 to 20 minutes about the solution: *How can you most easily …? What's the simplest way to …? What haven't you thought of yet? If there were a simple and elegant solution to this, what would it be? What things can you do? What things could you read? Which people can you ask for help?*

Once you truly analyze an obstacle, you see that it's not quite as big or impossible as you'd originally thought. As you start tapping into the other 90 percent of your brain, you'll discover solutions, and the process becomes fun!

But sometimes you just can't solve the issue on your own. That's the time to call in reinforcements, such as a life coach, a counselor, a therapist, or a trusted friend. They might be able to help you to get your feelings sorted and work through ways to improve the situation.

Plan for Follow-up Support

Hold on Tight to Your Support Network

If you reached goal weight with the help of a weight-loss coach, a sponsor, or an accountability partner, you shouldn't assume you can go it alone during the maintenance stage. Make sure you have a support system to guide you through the first year of maintenance.

If you didn't have a coach to kick-start your program, or if you did and your sessions have ended, consider joining group coaching to keep you motivated and accountable. You can also join a 12-step program or sign-up to my community at www.lindiscourtney.com. I can't say it enough—if you could do it on your own, you would have done it years ago. You must have help and support from others to achieve maintenance.

People who have access to experienced mentors and are surrounded by driven peers are much more likely to reach their goals than those without either. They figure things out faster, make fewer mistakes and are pushed to succeed by those around them. It's a formula for success.

Reaffirm Your Goals and Your Commitment to Change

Own Your Accomplishments

Just because you've achieved goal weight doesn't mean you should stop acknowledging your huge accomplishment. On a weekly basis, look back on your weight and food charts and acknowledge how far you've come. Keep track of the many smart choices you now make. You might even want to track how many days, week, or months that you've abstained from overeating. Be in awe of what you've learned and applied to your life. Continue to give yourself rewards for your ongoing success.

Relapse Is Normal

*"An ant will find a grain of sugar, if there is
a grain of sugar to be found."*
—Swami Shivapadananda

Once you've reached goal weight, you're not out of the danger zone. Relapse is a normal aspect of a major life change. There are degrees of relapse. A small-scale relapse would be knowingly eating much more than your stomach wanted or needed at a single meal. A large-scale relapse is when you overeat for several days in a row and start to gain back the weight you worked so hard to take off. Whether it's a small-scale or large-scale relapse, take some time to investigate. What triggered it? What were you thinking and feeling at the time? What can you do to avoid mistakes in the future?

If you experience a setback, the best solution is to start again with the preparation, action, or maintenance stages of behavioral change. You might want to reassess your resources and techniques. Do you have a support team in place? Reaffirm your motivation, your plan of action, and your commitment to your goals. Also, make plans for how you will deal with any future temptations.

Why Do You Fall Into Relapse?

Relapse is a good thing! What? Yes, because you're testing whether the old way is better than the new way. Even if you've been dropping weight and enjoying the new lifestyle, you might occasionally feel as if you're missing out on something. You see a huge cheesecake and you remember the good times you had eating massive amounts of cheesecake, how great it made you feel. You remember the good, but you forget all the things you hated about eating massive amounts of cheesecake. You hated to feel out of control, bloated, lethargic, and embarrassed that you couldn't stop at one piece, and you hated the headache and the low self-esteem that set in the following morning. You see the cake and remember only the good times. So you eat it—overeat it—and only then are you reminded why you wanted to change to begin with. You feel awful! So you tell yourself with renewed confidence, "The new way is the better way." You tested the old way and you choose the new way. It was a scientific experiment.

You know you're getting stronger when the periods between relapses grow longer and the actual relapse gets shorter. If you used to go off your eating plan every day and now it's just once every couple of weeks, that's major progress. **Instead of focusing on what you did wrong, focus on how far you've come.**

The most important thing to do after a relapse is to get back on track. Don't overcompensate or undercompensate; just work your plan as you normally would at the next meal. Fewer relapses lead to no relapses.

Identify Triggers That Lead to Relapse

A relapse typically doesn't come without warning. There are often small changes in your thinking or behavior that alert you to the fact that you're about to go off course. Here are a few of the common signs of a pending relapse:

Pride Goeth Before a Fall

Sometimes you become so overly elated about your accomplishments that you trick yourself into believing you're cured (though some experts believe no one is ever fully cured of an addiction to food, drugs or alcohol). If you believe you *are* cured or "normal," you might let your guard down. It's just like with an alcoholic who has gone 10 years without a drink and suddenly thinks, "I can handle it now." A food addict should always be on guard against this type of overconfidence.

Yes, you appear to be a normal eater to the outside world, and yes, it seems that you're cured, but that doesn't mean you should abandon the plan and habits that have cured you. The minute you indulge in random eating or, worse, disordered eating, you're back in a cycle of compulsive, out-of-control eating followed by self-badgering and restrictive eating.

Obsessing About Food

You might be losing weight steadily or even have reached the point of maintenance when suddenly you notice that you're spending a lot of time thinking, dreaming and obsessing about your former favorites. This can occur for a variety of reasons. Perhaps your meal plans have become monotonous and you miss the variety of your former days. Or certain problems have entered your life and you want to distract yourself with your drug of choice. Whatever the reason, the fact is that for the first time in a long time, triggers and cravings are starting to have power over you.

You'll have to play detective and ask yourself, "Why am I focusing so much on my former favorites? Why am I not more focused on achieving my purpose, strengthening relationships with others, or setting new goals for health and fitness?" If there are problems to work out, work them out. If your healthy meal plan is boring, spice it up. If you need support to stay on track, get help.

Remember that you get what you focus on. Focus on the problem and you drown in it. Focus on food and you eat it. Focus on an amazing body and an amazing life and you get them. What do you really want? At the end of the day, food is just food. It's fuel. It will never satisfy you like great relationships and meaningful work.

Feasible but No Longer Desirable?

Probably the biggest reason why people relapse during the maintenance stage is that even though they know that weight loss is feasible (they've done it!), they're no longer convinced it's desirable. They resort to their old habits of eating unhealthily because they conclude that it's more desirable to eat what they want when they want it than to be on a healthy eating plan. Despite the negative consequences, the food addict is tempted to return to his drug.

Sara was in the maintenance stage for 11 months, sustaining a 50-pound weight loss, when suddenly her willpower started to wane. She found herself secretly buying cookies and hiding them in her room. She'd eat them at night in bed while watching TV even though she knew the scale was on to her. Two extra pounds became 5 pounds, and 5 pounds became 10. Within three months, Sara had gained back 15 pounds. She was smart enough to ask for help.

"Losing weight was fun, but maintenance stinks," she said. "The meals are the same, the scale is the same, and my life is the same. Losing weight was motivating. Maintaining is boring."

In coaching, we took a closer look at Sara's life purpose (to be a teacher) and her values (education, family, and church), and I asked her if anything had changed.

"I don't want to be a teacher," she said. "I did substituting this summer and I hated it."

Bingo. Sara's life was in limbo. She didn't know what her purpose was, so, out of frustration, she'd gone back to the cookie jar. Through our sessions, she discovered new goals (find a husband, start a nonprofit), and that was enough to get her to lose the 15 pounds and stay there.

During the maintenance stage, people sometimes start to doubt that they deserve to be thin. "Who am I to be thin?" they think. "Why am I really doing this? Am I really going to be a thin person for the rest of my life?" If you have these thoughts, remind yourself that your disease is trying to trick you into going back to a life of chaotic eating and dieting. You don't want to face that turmoil and insecurity again. You don't want to return to an imprisoned life of pain and shame. You do deserve to be thin, and you do deserve to be free from the nightmare of food addiction.

HALT (hungry, angry, lonely, tired)

You'll be more susceptible to a relapse if you're hungry, angry, lonely, or tired. Instead of eating when you're vulnerable, do something to address the feeling.

If you feel more hunger than you're used to in the early stages of the new eating program, drink a glass or two of water when hunger strikes. Sometimes you're just thirsty. Another option is to do something that will make the time between meals go faster, such as running out for a quick shopping trip, watching an interesting show on TV, or calling a supportive friend. Once you've begun to lose regularly, you get more used to slight hunger between meals and you don't panic. You know it's part of losing weight.

When you're angry, you may fall into the routine of eating your anger away. What can you do instead? Can you write your anger thoughts into a journal? Can you assertively express your anger directly to the person who upset you? Can you call a friend or a family member to hash it out?

Eating when we're lonely only makes us lonelier. Food addicts have a history of keeping to themselves. They like isolation (to eat alone, to be ashamed alone, to try to take control of their eating alone). To counter loneliness, you must get connected to a community of people who can relate to what you're going through. Twelve-step programs and online communities are good options. Other ways to tackle loneliness are to write in a journal, start blogging, or read spiritually uplifting books that give you a better mind-set. I like to read the Bible or other Christian literature and take comfort in the fact that God is always there.

If you're tired, sleep! Take a nap or go to bed early. Studies have found that people who sleep eight to 10 hours a night are less prone to obesity than those who sleep less than eight hours. Sometimes we even eat to stay awake! How silly. Just go to bed.

Relapse Attitudes and Behaviors to Watch Out For

The following attitudes or behaviors usually indicate that you're about to fall into a relapse.

- Preferring to eat alone

- Having the "this-is-not-enough" mentality

- Pushing foods on to others

- Snacking while preparing a meal

- Adding extra food after you've planned what you'll put on the plate

- Thinking you'll be okay once you reach goal weight

- Constantly thinking about what to eat or not eat

- Thinking, "This little extra doesn't make a difference"

- No longer trying to discover new and exciting healthy meal combinations

- No longer writing down your planned and unplanned eating

- No longer weighing yourself on a daily basis

Fight the Relapse Urge

Before You Take That First Bite

Students do fire drills to practice exiting the scene of danger so that when a major crisis occurs, they know what to do. You should do the same in regard to avoiding a major relapse. I recommend that you create a clear-cut intervention plan on paper so that when a trigger situation strikes, you know what to do. Here are a few possibilities, but please create ones that will work for you.

- Get out of the area of danger (the kitchen, the ice cream store, the all-you-can-eat buffet line).

- Tell yourself, "I am a food addict. Food may be tempting, but nothing tastes as good as thin feels."

- Call a friend/sponsor/weight-loss coach or log in to your online community and start writing.

- Go for a walk and get some fresh air.

- Drink a glass or two of water. It cleanses and fills you.

- Read the list of accomplishments in your journal.

- Write in your journal how you're feeling and try to understand what triggered the craving.

- Ask yourself, "Do I want to feed the disease or my recovery?"

- Ask yourself, "Do I want to be overweight and out of control again?"

- Repeat a famous quote, Bible verse, or slogan that keeps you focused. For example: "Short-term indulgence is long-term agony."

- Read a chapter of a book on food-addiction recovery.

- Write the thoughts that are tempting you and then rewrite new thoughts that put you in a position of power and control. Use intentional thinking. What result do you want?

What else can you add to the list above that would work for you?

Recognize and Fulfill the True Underlying Urge

If you have a relapse urge that won't go away with one of the intervention plans above, you need to ask yourself what feeling you're looking to achieve by eating a particular food.

Can you find a better way to create that feeling?

Let's say you've just had one of the worst days of your life. You're down and depressed. You can't think about anything other than Haagen-Dazs Rocky Road ice cream, though you know that if you buy it, you'll eat the whole thing and feel sick to your stomach. What feeling do you hope to achieve by eating an entire container of Haagen-Dazs Rocky Road ice cream? The likely answer: drugged out, tired, relaxed, numb and secure.

Hmmmm. How can you get that same feeling without food (or illegal drugs!)? You jot down five alternative activities and choose to do the one that will give you what you really need.

- Go to sleep

- Rent a relaxing movie and curl up on the coach with a cozy blanket and pillow

- Listen to a relaxation CD that practically puts you to sleep

- Read a comforting book that inspires and feeds your soul

- Make chicken noodle soup for dinner

Pursue Your Purpose With a Vengeance

When you started on your journey of achieving your purpose and pursuing your goals, you were highly enthusiastic. The possibilities were endless, and motivation was at an all-time high. After a few weeks or months, however, it's easy to lose steam as doubts begin to arise. "Can I really achieve my life purpose?" you might ask yourself. "What if I never succeed?"

If you doubt your ability to achieve your goals in life, you may become dismayed and let that derail your eating. Rather than relapse into an eating frenzy, take steps to achieve your all-important life goals.

Below is a list of positive activities that will keep you out of the kitchen and passionate about your purpose:

- **Make a list about your purpose.** Brainstorm about the next steps you'll take to achieve your purpose. Who will you contact next? What will you research this week? Who can give you advice for this phase of the project? What can you read to prepare yourself for the next steps?

- **Brainstorm about yourself.** Build your self-esteem for this crucial next phase by focusing on all your strengths and past successes. You can draw a timeline from birth to the present and record every event you're proud of. Write down which strengths enabled you to succeed at particular times in life. You can also jot down all the characteristics you like about yourself, such as your great listening skills, your compassion for others and your contagious smile. Once it's all on paper, you'll see that you have a lot to offer the world.

- **Read inspiring quotes.** Sometimes just one quote can hit the nail on the head and get your heart and mind back on track and even catapult you further. If there isn't one quote that speaks to your current situation, write your own.

- **Cut out of magazines.** Cut out phrases or pictures that represent the new you. Perhaps it's a pretty beach house that you will one day enjoy with your family, or a Nike "just do it" advertisement that illustrates your future physical shape and stamina. You can also cut out pictures of people you'll help once you're living out your purpose. What type of people are they? What do they look like? Feel the urgency of their need for you to pursue your purpose so that you can be a blessing to them.

- **Listen to uplifting music.** We often have Christian children's music on in our car, and even when I'm driving alone, I sometimes play those CDs to keep me joyful. Find music that cheers you up and reminds you that you're never alone.

- **Read Inspirational books.** You can ensure success by recharging your mind on a daily basis. Get some spiritual refreshment for your soul in the morning and evening. You can do this by reading your own inspirational notes, pages from this book, the Bible, or 12-step literature. Reading the stories of others who have achieved similar feats will encourage you. Reading renews the mind, washes out old thoughts and replaces them with inspiring ones. Please see the Appendix for a recommended-reading list.

- **Create a strategy poster to keep you on target.** When I was about to write my first book, I created a huge poster with deadlines and key steps that I hung in my living room, much to my family's surprise. This little act helped me to focus, and it also made me accountable to my family, who saw very clearly what I needed to do and by when.

- **Buy uplifting and inspiring posters.** Posters depicting people pushing themselves, such as mountain climbers and runners, can remind you to press on and go for the gold. You can even post a sign expressing a sentiment you've written yourself, such as "I can do it!"

- **Do something refreshing.** If you think about your food plan or your life plan too much, you can lose your spontaneity and creativity. Take a break from everything by doing something refreshing, childlike or just plain silly. Drive to the beach and put your feet in the sand, ride a roller coaster and scream your head off, or just take a long brisk walk and notice the leaves, the clouds and the sounds of nature.

Bounce Back After Relapse

Next Meal Back on Track

There's only one way to bounce back after a relapse. Stop immediately and get back to planned eating. Don't eat less or more the day after. Just go right back to the food program. If you can't get back on track, get help one of these ways:

- Hire a weight-loss coach

- Join a 12-step group and get a sponsor

- Join an online community and get a "buddy" to hold you accountable

It's is also advisable to ask yourself:

- What or where was the trigger that set you off?

- What was the thought process you had after the trigger?

- What emotions did you feel after you zeroed in on your proposed action?

- How did you feel when you were eating?

- How did you feel when you were finished eating?

- How did you feel the day after?

- What did the scale say? How did that make you feel?

- What can you do next time to avoid reacting negatively to the trigger?

- What were the major causes of your previous relapses? Was this one similar?

- What specific action-oriented processes can you use to counter the situations and emotions that threaten to lead to relapse in the future?

- Can you tolerate a little slip without falling into a major relapse? (A slip is a minor incident of unplanned eating at a meal).

- Do you want to go back to your addiction or back to recovery?

Learn From the Relapse

If for some reason you do overeat, please sit down with pen and paper and write how you feel afterward. You'll want to read this the next time you even think about overeating!

For example: "Today I ate everything I could find in the house—pizza, chips, cookies, cheese—and then I even drove to McDonald's. I feel awful. I feel overweight, ugly, and out of control. Why did I do that? I hate the feeling of being out of control. I love when I'm eating healthy. Eating all that food didn't even satisfy me. It just made me sadder, and I felt more empty and alone than ever. I am not going to do this again. I am writing this down so that I can remember how horrible it feels to overeat. This is a part of my past life. I have a new life, and overeating just doesn't fit into it. I've learned from this mistake and I won't repeat it."

The next time the urge to go way off course strikes, read what you've written and ask yourself, "Is it worth it?" You'll probably say no and go do something valuable with your time, money and energy.

What Would You Do Next Time?
(Rehearse Re-patterning)

Writing down what we would do differently next time can help us to learn from our mistakes—we're so much wiser after the fact. If you overate at a company party when you found yourself standing in the buffet line with so many yummy choices, what could you do if the situation arose again tomorrow?

You could rehearse re-patterning by imagining yourself at the buffet line and saying to yourself:

- "First, I would take a quick walk around the buffet table to see what my options are."

- "Then I would grab three items (chicken, vegetables and a potato). I wouldn't even look at the dessert table. Coffee would be my dessert."

- "If anyone asked me if I wanted to go up for seconds or dessert, I would say, 'No thanks, I'm so full!'"

Get into the habit of mentally rehearsing re-patterning after an incident so that the new patterns become ingrained in your mind and body.

Go Easy on Yourself

The last thing you want to do after a relapse is beat yourself up. People who have struggled with their weight have been beating themselves up for years, and that hasn't been very helpful. Instead of focusing on the relapse, focus on what you've accomplished.

You can say the following, for example. "OK, so I fell into a minor relapse yesterday, but if I look at how far I've come, I can really be proud of myself. So far I've lost _____ pounds. I used to overeat several times a day/week, but now I'm only doing this once a week/month/etc. I've come so far in changing my behaviors that this little slip isn't going to be a major setback. I needed to test my old ways to see if they were worth going back to. They aren't. I'm much happier engaging in my new, healthier ways. I will achieve my target weight of ___."

6
STAGE

Termination:

"I Am Forever Thin!"

CHARACTERISTICS OF TERMINATION	HELPFUL STRATEGIES
• Food addiction is no longer a problem, temptation or threat • You have complete confidence that you will be a normal eater without relapsing • You won the battle!	• Finish-line exhilaration • A new attitude and self-image • Ingrained habits • Self-enhancing, purpose-driven living

"There is one quality that one must possess to win,
and that is definiteness of purpose, the knowledge of what
one wants, and a burning desire to possess it."

—Napoleon Hill

Characteristics of Termination

Termination is the ultimate goal in the change process. As a recovered food addict, you no longer see food as a temptation or a threat. You have complete confidence that you can cope with life without fear of a major relapse. You experience zero temptation to embrace your former ways and have developed new patterns for maintaining a healthy, normal and stress-free relationship with food.

Finish-Line Exhilaration

Reaching goal weight is like running a marathon. At first you aren't sure whether you can do it, but you eventually get going and your faith in yourself increases. Then you hit a wall and think, "Should I quit?" No! You press on. The pain is excruciating, and the battle between sticking with it and throwing in the towel throws you into emotional turmoil, but just when you're about to give up, you see the finish line in the distance. Then you know it. You can do it. You've *been* doing it. You're almost there. Your pace quickens, you get a second wind, and you fly the rest of the way. You cross the finish line. You did it!

Reaching goal weight is an exhilarating feeling of satisfaction and achievement. It's like being on top of the world, and it will rank up there as one of your most amazing accomplishments in life. Every time you look in the mirror, you're reminded of your victory. Congratulate yourself. Revel in the joy. Give praise to your efforts, commitment, strength and fortitude. Your persistence gives hope to others.

A New Attitude and Self-Image

You've crossed the finish line, and your body isn't the only thing that's changed. You've changed in many ways. Over the past few months, your self-esteem and your overall outlook on life have evolved. You have an inspiring new attitude and self-image to go with that new body. You have renewed faith in yourself and what the world has to offer you. You're embracing the person within you who's been dying to come out all these years. You're confident and assertive, and you radiate joy.

Don't be modest and keep your wisdom and enthusiasm to yourself. Share it. Be proud of what you've learned and accomplished. Don't be surprised if people push you into the spotlight because they're excited about your remarkable change and they want to learn from it.

Ingrained Habits (No More Temptations!)

You got to this amazing stage in your life because you learned to develop healthy new habits and patterns that work to your advantage. You're no longer tempted by unhealthy food or see former favorites as threats, but that doesn't mean you can drop the routines that got you where you are. Most likely, you'll continue to do the following:

- Exercise three to five days a week

- Be mindful, conscious and aware of what you're eating (some people keep a food journal for one to three years after losing a considerable amount of weight)

- Focus on the continuous journey of finding healthy new foods to incorporate into your meals

- Keep up with your community of recovered food addicts and give back by encouraging others

- Continue to journal your thoughts and the results that you want your thoughts to deliver.

Purpose-Driven Living

Now that eating properly and exercising are second nature to you, it's time to set new milestones for other important goals in your life (career, finances, relationships, etc.). Everything you learned along the road to achieving your weight goals can be applied to reaching these other important goals. This continuous pursuit of goals is a major aspect of joyful living.

As you carry out your purpose and experience victory in your weight-loss efforts, your life will start to attract quite a bit of attention. People will ask you about your transformation. What happened? What are you doing? What are you eating? Why are you smiling all the time? Are you in love?

Since we've discovered the secret to a joyful life, it becomes our great privilege and responsibility to share the good news. Many of your family members, co-workers, neighbors, and acquaintances are searching and longing for purpose, meaning and inner peace. Even those who appear to have it all may need someone to guide them. As you grow and develop in your confidence and purpose, you will continue to be a vehicle for hope and inspiration. Your life and your actions will be so significant, so powerful, so contagious that you can affect all the people you come into contact with in this lifetime.

Thank you for undergoing this exciting journey of reaching goal weight while pursuing your purpose! I look forward to hearing how you're using your abilities and passions to affect the world. I hope you will teach others to answer their hearts' call and live out their dreams. I pray that your life will be a continuous and faithful blessing to others.

Be sure to drop me a line and let me know how this book has benefited you (info@lindiscourtney.com).

Appendix

Inspirational Quotes

"By recording your dreams and goals on paper, you set in motion the process of becoming the person you most want to be. Put your future in good hands—your own."
—Mark Victor Hansen

"First say to yourself what you would be; and then do what you have to do."
—Epictetus

"One needs something to believe in, something for which one can have whole-hearted enthusiasm. One needs to feel that one's life has meaning, that one is needed in this world."
—Hanna Senesh

"Many people have a wrong idea of what constitutes true happiness. It is not attained through self-gratification, but through fidelity to a worthy purpose."
—Helen Keller

"All men should strive to learn before they die, what they are running from, and to, and why."
—James Thurber

"I have one life and one chance to make it count for something. ... I'm free to choose what that something is, and the something I've chosen is my faith. Now, my faith goes beyond theology and religion and requires considerable work and effort. My faith demands—this is not optional—my faith demands that I do whatever I can, wherever I am, whenever I can, for as long as I can with whatever I have to try to make a difference."
—Jimmy Carter

"Give yourself an even greater challenge than the one you are trying to master and you will develop the powers necessary to overcome the original difficulty."
—William J. Bennett, The Book of Virtues

"Whatever you can do, or dream you can, begin it. Boldness has genius, magic, and power in it."
—Johann Wolfgang Von Goethe

"For I know the plans I have for you," declares the Lord, "plans to prosper you and not to harm you, plans to give you hope and a future. "
—Jeremiah 29:11 New International Version (NIV)

Books for Recovery

Abstinence: Members of Overeaters Anonymous Share Their Experience, Strength, and Hope, by Overeaters Anonymous. 1994

Changing for Good: A Revolutionary Six-Stage Program for Overcoming Bad Habits and Moving Your Life Positively Forward, by James O. Prochaska. William Morrow Paperbacks, 1995

Conquer Your Food Addiction, by Caryl Ehrlich. Free Press, 2003

Feel the Fear and Do It Anyway, 20th-anniversary edition, by Susan Jeffers. Ballantine Books, 2006

From the First Bite: A Complete Guide to Recovery From Food Addiction, by Kay Sheppard. HCI, 2000

If I Am So Smart, Why Can't I Lose Weight? by Brooke Castillo. BookSurge Publishing, 2006

Life's Healing Choices: Freedom from Your Hurts, Hang-ups, and Habits, by John Baker. Howard Books, 2007

Self-Coach 101, by Brooke Castillo. Futures Unlimited Coaching, 2008

Taming Your Gremlin: A Surprisingly Simple Method for Getting Out of Your Own Way, revised edition, by Rick Carlson. Quill, 2003

Celebrate Recovery Bible. Zondervan, 2007

The Twelve Steps and Twelve Traditions of Overeaters Anonymous, by Overeaters Anonymous

Voices of Recovery: A Daily Reader, by Overeaters Anonymous

Self-Help Groups

Overeaters Anonymous

Overeaters Anonymous offers a program of recovery from compulsive eating using the Twelve Steps and Twelve Traditions of OA. Worldwide meetings and other tools provide a fellowship of experience, strength and hope where members respect one another's anonymity. OA charges no dues or fees; it is self-supporting through member contributions. OA is not just about weight loss, weight gain, maintenance, obesity, and diets. It addresses physical, emotional, and spiritual well-being. It is not a religious organization and does not promote any particular diet. Find a meeting in person, online, or over the telephone by visiting their website www.oa.org.

Food Addicts Anonymous

Food Addicts Anonymous is an organization that believes that food addiction is a biochemical disorder that occurs at a cellular level and therefore cannot be cured by willpower or therapy alone. This 12-step program believes that food addiction can be managed by abstaining from (eliminating) addictive foods, following a program of sound nutrition (a food plan), and working the 12 steps of the program. FAA is self-supporting. No dues or fees are required for membership, only a desire to stop eating addictive foods. You can review the recommended food plan and find out about meeting times at www.foodaddictsanonymous.org.

Celebrate Recovery

Celebrate Recovery is a 12-step, Christ-centered ministry designed to help those struggling with hurts, hang-ups, and habits by showing them the loving power of Jesus Christ through the recovery process. More than 700,000 people have gone through the Celebrate Recovery program in more than 17,000 churches worldwide. To learn more about this program or to find a group in your area, visit www.celebraterecovery.com.

Exercise DVDs

Below is a list of DVDs ranging from beginner to advanced levels. Check out the product description on their websites, so that you can choose the ones that are best for your level of fitness and personal goals.

- Beachbody Insanity DVD. www.beachbody.com

- Beachbody TurboFile Greatest HIITs: 20 Minute High Intensity Workout DVD. www.beachbody.com

- Beachbody P90X. www.beachbody.com

- Beachbody 10-Minute Trainer. www.beachbody.com

- Billy Blanks' Tae Bo: The Ultimate Collection. www.Billyblanks. com

- Fat-Burning Kickboxing Workout for Dummies. www.amazon.com

- 5 Really Big Miles DVD (walking). www.walkathome.com

- Leslie Sansone Walk Away the Pounds - Walk and Kick DVD ~ Leslie Sansone

- Ministry of Sound : The Ultimate Workout—Pump It Up, Burn It, Lose It. www.ministryofsound.com/shop/fitness

- The Ultimate Zumba Fitness DVD Experience. www.zumbafitness. com

- 10 Minute Solution: Kickbox Bootcamp. www.the10minutesolution. com

- 10 Minute Solution: Rapid Results Pilates. www. the10minutesolution.com

Bibliography

[1] Prochaska, James O. *Changing for Good: A Revolutionary Six-Stage Program for Overcoming Bad Habits and Moving Your Life Positively Forward.* New York: William Morrow Paperbacks, 1995

[2] U.S. Department of Health and Human Services, National Institutes of Health, National Health, Lung and Blood Institute. "The Clinical Guidelines on the Identification, Evaluation and Treatment of Overweight and Obesity in Adults: Evidence Report." NH pub. No. 98-4083, September 1998

[3] U.S. Department of Health and Human Services. "At-a-glance: A Fact Sheet for Professionals. Physical Activity Guidelines for Americans." <http://www.health.gov/paguidelines/factsheetprof.aspx>

[4] Mayo Clinic. "The Daily Caloric Consumption Chart for Women." In Mayo Clinic Report 163 (1998). *American Journal of Clinical Nutrition* 44:1-19

[5] "Cheesecake-eating rats and the question of food addiction." In *Nature Neuroscience* 13:529–531, 2010

[6] Gearhardt A.N ., Corbin W.R., Brownell KD. "Preliminary validation of the Yale Food Addiction Scale." In *Appetite* 52(2):430-6, 2009. Epub 2008

[7] Corbin, Brownell. "Yale Food Addiction Scale." 2009. http://www.resoundinghealth.com/static/Yale_Food_Addiction_Scale.pdf.

[8] Pollan, Michael. *In Defense of Food: An Eater's Manifesto.* London: Penguin Press, 2008

[9,10] Ibid

[11] Covey, Stephen. *Seven Habits of Highly Effective People*. Fireside, 1989

[12] "Psychology of success: Broncos players use visualization skills." *The Gazette,* 2006. http://www.highbeam.com/doc/1P2-3699711.html

[13] Chan, Amanda. "Diet Soda Linked to Weight Gain." *Huffington Post*, posted June 29, 2011. http://www.huffingtonpost.com/2011/06/29/diet-soda-weight-gain_n_886409.html

[14] Park, Alice. "Can Sugar Substitutes Make You Fat?" In *Time Health*, Feb. 10, 2008. http://www.time.com/time/health/article/0,8599,1711763,00.html

[15] Moritz, Andreas. "Diet Sweeteners Can Make You Sick and Fat." On *Natural News.com*, March 2008. http://www.naturalnews.com/022785.html

[16] Kirchheimer, Sid. "Too Much White Bread Giving You a Big Belly? Eat More Fiber-Filled Foods Like Fruits, Vegetables, and Whole Grains." On *WebMD,* Aug. 4, 2004 http://www.webmd.com/diet/news/20040803/too-much-white-bread-giving-you-big-belly

[17] Jeffers, Susan. Feel the Fear and Do It Anyway. New York: Ballantine Books, 1988

[18] Ibid

[19] Carlson, Rich. Taming Your Gremlin: A Surprisingly Simple Method for Getting Out of Your Own Way, revised edition. Quill, 2003

[20] Covey, Stephen. Seven Habits of Highly Effective People. New York: Fireside, 1989

[21] Ibid

About the Author

Lindis Courtney has over 20 years of experience in motivating and inspiring people to achieve their personal and business goals. In 2009, after two decades of successfully climbing corporate ladders in leadership positions in the United States and Europe, Lindis chose to pursue her true passion: serving as an inspirational weight-loss coach and writer. She has an undergraduate degree from the State University of New York at Binghamton. In addition, she has studied theology at Talbot Theological Seminary, psychology at Chapman University, and coaching at the International Coaching Academy.

Today, Lindis runs a private weight-loss coaching practice in Norway, where she lives with her husband and five children. Join Lindis' community at www.lindiscourtney.com.

www.ingramcontent.com/pod-product-compliance
Lightning Source LLC
Chambersburg PA
CBHW070010300526
45794CB00001B/259